A GLOSSARY OF

MEDICAL PHYSIOLOGY

Dr. Ginsburg,
With best wishes
from the author
Enjoy the book!

Patrick
7/17/12

A GLOSSARY OF

MEDICAL PHYSIOLOGY

A COMPANION TEXT FOR STUDENTS IN THE MEDICAL AND HEALTH SCIENCES AND HEALTH CARE PROFESSIONALS

ANTHONY B. EBEIGBE
PATRICK N. OLOMU

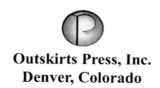

Outskirts Press, Inc.
Denver, Colorado

A Glossary of Medical Physiology
A Companion Text for Students in the Medical and Health Sciences and Health Care Professionals
All Rights Reserved.
Copyright © 2011 Anthony B. Ebeigbe and Patrick N. Olomu
v6.0

Outskirts Press, Inc.
http://www.outskirtspress.com

ISBN: 978-1-4327-7705-0

Library of Congress Control Number: 2010904697

Outskirts Press and the "OP" logo are trademarks belonging to Outskirts Press, Inc.

PRINTED IN THE UNITED STATES OF AMERICA

Notice

The authors and publisher have made every effort to ensure that the information in this text is in accordance with current knowledge and standards accepted at the time of publication. Medical and health sciences are ever-changing fields. As new research and clinical experience broaden our knowledge, changes in clinical practice and drug therapy are required. The authors and publisher do not guarantee that the information in this work will always be accurate and they disclaim all responsibility for results obtained from use of the information contained herein. Also, treatment modalities and drug therapy can change, not only from new research, but also from government regulations. Readers are therefore encouraged to cross-check information in this book with other sources.

This book is dedicated to my father, for the exemplary principles of his life.

A.B.E

To V.K.O, my late mother, for nurturing me in those early years. Your love, strength, and example will forever be cherished. To Neeta and Megan, for your unyielding support despite the many hours and late nights devoted to working on this book.

P.N.O

Contents

Foreword

A Glossary of Medical Physiology by Anthony Ebeigbe and Patrick Olomu represents another significant contribution to the literature for the understanding of concepts in medical physiology. Physiology as a subject is the essential framework for subsequent understanding of clinical medicine and the medical sciences. This subject area has been the focus of many historical standard texts which have been of use over the years in many institutions both locally and abroad. However, the present text differs in its approach to the presentation of the subject. It has adopted an alphabetical treatment approach to the contents and subject matter which makes it very easy to use and easy to assimilate.

The content of this book, despite its brevity, underscores its comprehensive approach to the topics that are treated which cover the whole spectrum of medical physiology. These topics are explained in simple, yet scientifically explicit terms as to avoid any ambiguity. The explanation of each glossary term is very precise and concise. The broad areas covered make this text a very compelling and useful read, despite its size. It is almost tempting to conclude that this book is in itself a total treatment of the subject matter. However, it will still be necessary for users of the book to read it along with any of the various standard texts that are available.

The book will be very useful to a wide audience, not only to medical and dental students, but also students in other medical sciences such as pharmacology, physiology, physiotherapy, radiography, medical laboratory sciences, nursing, and optometry among others. Additionally, this will be a very useful desk-top text for all practicing medical and dental practitioners as well as those preparing for the Primary examinations of the various Postgraduate Medical Colleges.

The lucidness and simplicity of this book make it a very highly recommended text. Its currency of contents will enable it to also have a long shelf life. The authors are to be congratulated for this unique and landmark work, especially as they have made available to the users, the benefits of their long and distinguished experience as medical educators and researchers.

Professor Olusoga A. Sofola, MBBS, PhD, FAS (Nigeria)
Professor of Physiology
College of Medicine, University of Lagos
Lagos, Nigeria

Preface

A Glossary of Medical Physiology is a new and unique addition to the broad field of medical physiology. Unlike other well recognized textbooks in medical physiology, an alphabetical keyword approach that addresses the core concepts in medical physiology has been adopted. Key concepts that are required knowledge for students and practitioners in the medical and health sciences have been carefully selected. The list of over **1600** entries covers core areas of medical physiology, biochemistry, molecular biology, pharmacology, immunology, and not least, medical history. Additionally, the clinical correlations of many of the keywords have been emphasized thus putting them in a clear and concise clinical context. Also, many of the entries have been extensively cross-referenced in an effort to enhance the book's educational value.

This *Glossary* would be an invaluable reading guide and a quick review source for students in the basic sciences and those preparing for the basic science component of their professional examinations. For health care practitioners, especially those preparing for postgraduate examinations, the *Glossary* provides a quick and refreshing review of the essentials of medical physiology and related subjects. The book has been designed to be of tremendous benefit to students and practitioners in the medical, dental, pharmaceutical, nursing and other allied health sciences.

Professor Anthony B. Ebeigbe, PhD

Patrick N. Olomu, MD, FRCA

November 2010

Acknowledgements

I am grateful to Miss Philomena Adozi for secretarial assistance and to Drs. Chukwuemeka Nwokocha and Ifedayo Ajayi for their valuable comments and suggestions. Much of this work was done during my sabbatical appointment as the Richard A. Bernstein Chair at the University of Maryland, Eastern Shore, MD, USA.

A.B.E.

My gratitude is owed first and foremost to Professor Anthony Ebeigbe, my uncle, teacher, and mentor, for inviting me to join him in this wonderful and very rewarding pursuit. I hope that my daily application of sound physiologic principles that you so elegantly taught will be a source of pride and fulfillment to you. To my father, a doctor of soil chemistry, for imbuing me with the love of science. My thanks also go to my teachers at the University of Ibadan College of Medicine for guiding me through the rigorous path to a successful career in medicine. Many accolades to Alethea Kalogiros and Roxana Pickering for their secretarial assistance and to Radu Pop for bringing the illustrations in this book to life.

P.N.O.

About the Authors

Dr. Anthony B. Ebeigbe is a Professor of Physiology at the College of Medical Sciences, University of Benin (UNIBEN), Benin City, Nigeria, where he has been involved in the teaching of Medical Physiology at both the undergraduate and postgraduate levels as well as research for over thirty years. He obtained the B.Sc. (Hons.) degree in Physiology from the University of Ibadan, Nigeria and his Ph.D. degree from the University of Glasgow, UK. He has held several important university positions, including: Head of Physiology Department, Dean at the College of Medicine, Edo State University, Nigeria and Provost of the College of Health Sciences at UNIBEN. He was, until recently, the Director of International Programs at UNIBEN and has been Visiting Professor to a number of institutions in Europe and the USA. Professor Ebeigbe is also the recipient of numerous honors and awards. He is a former Fulbright Scholar/Visiting Research Scientist at the University of Michigan Medical School, Ann Arbor, USA, Chairman of the Research Committee at UNIBEN, Editor-in-Chief of the Nigerian Journal of Physiological Sciences and was the Richard A. Bernstein Professor at the Department of Natural Sciences, University of Maryland Eastern Shore, USA. He is also a former President of the Physiological Society of Nigeria and currently, the Executive Director of Global Educational Initiative for Nigeria – a higher education non-governmental organization. Professor Ebeigbe is a member of many professional associations including: The Physiological Society of the United Kingdom, British Pharmacological Society and the American Physiological Society. His area of specialization is cardiovascular physiology and pharmacology where he has employed various techniques, including: Electron microscopy, radioisotope $^{45}Ca^{2+}$ fluxes as well as in vitro tension measurements on vascular smooth muscles, to elucidate the cellular mechanisms of action of a wide variety of vasoactive agents, in health and in disease states.

Dr. Patrick N. Olomu is an Assistant Professor of Anesthesiology and a pediatric anesthesiologist at the University of Texas Southwestern Medical Center and Children's Medical Center Dallas, Dallas, USA. He obtained his medical degree from the University of Ibadan College Of Medicine. He started his anesthesiology training at the University of Benin Teaching Hospital (UBTH) and continued his residency training in Hannover, Germany, the United Kingdom, and the United States. Upon completion of his anesthesiology residency in Chicago, Dr. Olomu completed a fellowship in Pediatric Anesthesia at Harvard Medical School and Children's Hospital Boston. He is a Diplomate of the American Board of Anesthesiology, Fellow of the Royal College of Anaesthetists of the United Kingdom and a Fellow of the American Academy of Pediatrics. He also has a Diploma in Anesthesiology from the University of Benin, Nigeria. Dr. Olomu was a recipient of the Federal Government of Nigeria Merit Award for outstanding academic achievement in medical school as well as the German Academic Exchange Award. Dr. Olomu has lectured extensively on various aspects of pediatric anesthesia and pediatric airway management to physicians, dentists, nurses and paramedical staff. His areas of interest are high-risk neonatal and pediatric anesthesia, advanced pediatric airway management and applied medical physiology and pharmacology. He has authored publications in the areas of pediatric airway management, anesthetic monitoring equipment, and general anesthetic management and practice.

A

A-Band

A region of the myofibril containing thick (myosin) filaments. *Also see thick filaments.*

Abdomen

The part of the trunk between the diaphragm and pelvis.

Abductor

A muscle that moves a body part away from the median plane. *Also see adductor.*

ABO System

System of classification for red blood cell (RBC) antigens. Based on presence of antigens on the red blood cell surface. There are four distinct blood group types: A, B, AB, and O. Figure shows specific antibody carried by each blood group type. Individuals with type AB blood have A and B antigens on their RBC and no antibodies. They can receive blood from all other groups and are called "universal recipients." Type O individuals have no antigens, can give blood to all other groups and are called "universal donors." The ABO system is the basis for blood typing and cross-matching to assure compatibility prior to a blood transfusion.

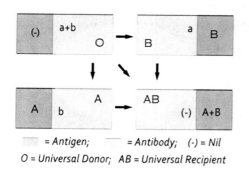

= Antigen; = Antibody; (-) = Nil
O = Universal Donor; AB = Universal Recipient

Abscess

A localized collection of pus in a cavity or space.

Absorption

The process by which molecules are transported across epithelial membranes into body fluids.

Acalculia

The inability to perform simple problems of arithmetic.

Accommodation

The automatic adjustment of the focal length of the lens, which results in the image of objects from varying distances coming into focus on the retina.

Acetyl CoA

Acetyl coenzyme A. It combines with choline to produce acetylcholine. It is the precursor of HMG-CoA, which is vital for cholesterol and ketone synthesis. *Also see HMG-CoA.*

Acetylcholine (Ach)

An acetic acid ester of choline. Acetylcholine is a local hormone and neurotransmitter in somatic motor nerves and parasympathetic nerve fibers. It was originally called *vagusstoff* by Otto Loewi in 1921 because vagal stimulation releases the chemical substance which slowed the heart. Acts on two receptor subtypes: nicotinic and muscarinic (many subtypes of the muscarinic receptor have been described -M1, M2 and M3). Nicotinic receptors are located postsynaptically on:

- Autonomic ganglia – when stimulated, produce excitatory postsynaptic potentials.
- Skeletal muscle motor endplates – stimulation causes depolarization resulting in endplate potentials (EPPs)
- Adrenal medulla – when stimulated, results in release of stored catecholamines.

Muscarinic receptors are located on effector organs with postganglionic cholinergic innervation e.g.

- Exocrine glands – stimulation causes increased secretion, heart – stimulation causes decrease in rate and force of contraction.
- Smooth muscle – stimulation causes contraction of intestinal smooth muscles

Depolarizing muscle relaxants such as succinylcholine potentiate the effects of Ach resulting in non-responsiveness. Non-depolarizing relaxants produce competitive inhibition of Ach at postjunctional sites of the neuromuscular junction. Anticholinergic agents have wide clinical uses in the treatment and prevention of bradycardia, as antisialologues (dry secretions), bronchodilation, and reversal of neuromuscular block (block the muscarinic effects of anticholinesterases such as neostigmine). *Otto Loewi – German physiologist. Also see autonomic receptors, cholinergic receptors, and atropine.*

Acetylcholinesterase

An enzyme located in the postsynaptic membrane of the neuromuscular junction that inactivates acetylcholine by converting it to choline and acetic acid. Anticholinesterases potentiate the effects of acetylcholine. Neostigmine and physostigmine are commonly used anticholinesterases. The former is used to reverse non-depolarizing muscle relaxants. Pyridostigmine, another anticholinesterase, is used for the treatment of myasthenia gravis. *Also see acetylcholine, atropine, and myasthenia gravis.*

Acid-base balance

The balance between acidity and alkalinity; required to keep the blood pH at a normal level of 7.40 ±0.05. *Also see pH.*

Acidosis

A state in which arterial pH falls below 7.35. In primary *metabolic acidosis*, the arterial CO_2 changes in the same direction as the pH ($\downarrow$ pH and $\downarrow$ $PaCO_2$).

In primary *respiratory acidosis*, the $PaCO_2$ changes in the opposite direction as the pH ($\downarrow$ pH and $\uparrow$ $PaCO_2$). Alveolar hypoventilation from various causes is the most common cause. *Also see pH, Alkalosis, buffer, and Henderson-Hasselbalch equation.*

Acinar cells

Cells present in exocrine glands, responsible for secretions; they are enclosed by myoepithelial cells which, upon contraction, squeeze the secretions through the ducts.

Acromegaly

A chronic disease of adults caused by over secretion of growth hormone from the pituitary. It is associated with enlargement of bones of the hands, jaw, face, and feet as well as other systemic complications. *Also see gigantism and growth hormone.*

ACTH

Adrenocorticotropic hormone. A polypeptide hormone secreted by the anterior pituitary; it stimulates the adrenal cortex to secrete adrenocortical steroids (mainly cortisol). High blood levels of corticosteroid decrease ACTH secretion by a negative feedback mechanism. Stress is a potent stimulus for ACTH secretion. It is also called corticotrophin.

Actin

A contractile protein of muscle cells; it exists in two forms: globular and fibrous. Actin, together with troponin and tropomyosin, make up the proteins of the thin filaments. *Also see myosin, thin, thick and intermediate filaments.*

Action Potential

Action potential is the sudden change in the membrane electrical activity of excitable tissues (nerve and muscle), associated with rapid reversal, and followed by reestablishment of the resting membrane potential. It is induced by a threshold (or greater) stimulus. The stimulus may be electrical, mechanical (pressure, touch, light) or chemical (smell, taste). The depolarization phase is due to increased permeability to Na+ while the repolarization phase is due to increase conductance of K^+. Action potentials demonstrate the "all-or-none" phenomenon. *Also see All-or-none-law and refractory period.*

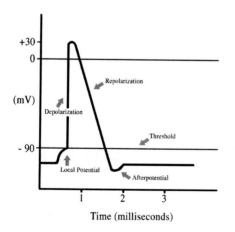

Nerve Action Potential

Active Immunity

A form of acquired immunity where the body produces its own antibodies against disease-producing antigens. Active immunity can be acquired in two ways: by vaccination or by contracting an infectious disease.

Active Transport

An energy-dependent movement of molecules or ions across cell membranes of epithelial cells by means of membrane carriers. The molecules or ions move uphill against a concentration gradient - electrical or pressure. There are two types of active transport (based on energy source): *primary active transport* – requires energy from ATP breakdown and *secondary active transport* – requires energy previously stored in transmembrane ionic concentration differences.

Activin

A plasma glycoprotein that stimulates the secretion of *follicle-stimulating hormone* by the pituitary gland.

Acuity

Sharpness or quality of a sensation.

Acute

Sharp, severe, having sudden onset, sharp rise and short course; lasting a short time; seriously demanding urgent attention.

Acute care

The phase of managing health problems that is conducted in a hospital on patients needing immediate or urgent medical attention.

Adaptation

The process by which a sense organ such as the eye, adjusts to varying stimulus intensities such as lighting conditions.

Addison's disease

Adrenocortical dysfunction resulting in both mineralocorticoid and glucocorticoid deficiency. Adrenal crisis is a life-threatening condition which requires immediate treatment with appropriate intravenous fluids and glucorticoids.

Adductor

A muscle that pulls a body part toward the median plane. *Also see abductor.*

Adenohypophysis

The anterior, glandular lobe of the pituitary gland. It comprises three major cell types:

- acidophils, which secrete growth hormone (GH) and prolactin (PRL)
- basophils, which secrete adrenocorticotropic hormone (ACTH), thyroid stimulating hormone (TSH), follicle

stimulating hormone (FSH) and luteinizing hormone (LH) and

- Chromophobes, which have few cytoplasmic granules, may have secretory activity.

Secretions of the anterior pituitary are controlled by hormones secreted by the hypothalamus. *Also see trophic hormones.*

Adenosine Triphosphate (ATP)

A nucleotide with three phosphate groups. Conversion of ATP to ADP and pyrophosphate provides energy for cellular processes.

Adenylate Cyclase

See Adenylyl cyclase.

Adenylyl Cyclase

An enzyme found in cell membranes that catalyzes the conversion of ATP to cyclic AMP and pyrophosphate (PPi). It is called adenylate cyclase or adenyl cyclase in older literature.

Adiadochokinesia

Inability to stop one movement and follow it immediately with movement in the opposite direction.

ADH

See antidiuretic hormone.

Adipose Tissue

A type of loose connective tissue composed of adipocytes (fat cells); it is located primarily in deep subcutaneous layers under the skin where it provides insulation. It also is found around internal organs where it provides a protective cushion reserve for nutrients.

ADP (Adenosine Diphosphate)

An ester of adenosine; in combination with inorganic phosphate, it is converted to ATP (adenosine triphosphate) for energy storage.

Adrenal Cortex

The outer part (cortex) of the adrenal gland; it is derived from the embryonic mesoderm. It has three distinct zones –an outer zona glomerulosa, an intermediate zona fasciculata, and an inner zona reticularis. The adrenal cortex secretes glucocorticoids, mineralocorticoids and sex steroids and the different layers exhibit some degree of specialization in the type of hormones they produce. Because of the important effects of these hormones on metabolism and fluid and electrolyte balance, the adrenal cortex is essential for survival. *Also see Addison's disease.*

Adrenal Medulla

The inner part of the adrenal gland that is derived from embryonic postganglionic sympathetic neurons.

Sympathetic stimulation of the adrenal medulla induces the release of epinephrine and norepinephrine (80:20 ratio) into the circulation. A *pheochromocytoma* is a secretory tumor of the adrenal medulla that produces severe cardiovascular effects, especially severe hypertension.

Adrenaline

Neurotransmitter substance or hormone produced by the adrenal medulla. Large amounts are released into the circulation during stress. Also called epinephrine.

Adrenergic Receptors

Receptors located on effector organs of the sympathetic nervous system. The two main types of adrenergic receptors are: α and β. Some organs have only alpha or beta receptors while others e.g. the heart, have both. The receptors are further divided into α_1, α_2, β_1, β_2 subtypes. Central nervous system α_2 receptors are inhibitory and decrease sympathetic output. The specific adrenergic agonists are norepinephrine and epinephrine, released from sympathetic postganglionic neurons and the adrenal medulla, respectively. The effects of stimulating adrenergic receptors include increase in the rate and force of contraction of the heart, vasoconstriction in the viscera and skin, glycogenolysis in the liver and bronchodilation. Because epinephrine has a greater effect on beta receptors, it has a more cardio-stimulating effect. Epinephrine is a weaker vasoconstrictor than norepinephrine since blood vessels contain mainly alpha receptors. Also, epinephrine causes a greater increase in general body metabolism. Antagonists at adrenergic receptors include Prazosin (α_1), Yohimbine (α_2), Propranolol (β_1, β_2). Adrenergic agonists and antagonists are widely used in clinical practice especially in the treatment cardiovascular diseases (hypertension, control of heart rate, and arrhythmias), asthma, and pain control. Clonidine is a centrally acting α_2 agonist that has wide clinical use in the treatment of hypertension and pain. Dexmedetomidine is a new, highly selective α_2 adrenergic agonist that exhibits sedative, analgesic, and anxiolytic properties. *Also see autonomic receptors, parasympathetic nervous system and catecholamines.*

Aerobic Capacity

Denotes the maximum rate of oxygen consumption (maximal oxygen uptake) by the body per unit time during intense exercise. It is a measure of cardio-respiratory fitness.

Affective Disorders   Psychiatric illnesses characterized mostly by mood abnormalities. The two principal categories are *mania* and *depression*. Many patients go through phases of both - manic depressive illness.

Afferent   Conveying or transmitting inward, toward center. Afferent neurons, for example, conduct impulses from the sense organs toward the central nervous system; afferent arterioles carry blood toward the glomerulus. *Also see efferent.*

Ageusia   *See Gustation.*

Agglutination   Clumping of red blood cells induced by specific chemical interaction between surface antigens and antibodies.

Agglutinin   An antibody that causes agglutination of a particular antigen, especially red blood cells or bacteria.

Agnosia   Failure to recognize familiar objects despite an intact sensory mechanism. May occur for any sensory modality.

Agranular leukocytes   Types of white blood cells (lymphocytes and monocytes) that contain small, poorly visible cytoplasmic granules.

Agraphia   Inability to express thoughts in writing.

Akinetic mutism   A condition of silent, alert-appearing, immobility that characterizes certain subacute or chronic states of altered consciousness. Sleep-wake cycles are retained, but no observable evidence of mental activity is evident; spontaneous motor activity is lacking; the individual appears to be aware but inactive. Exhibited by individuals with high brain stem lesions.

Albumin   A simple water-soluble protein produced in the liver; the major component of the plasma proteins. Cow (bovine) albumin is often used as an enzyme stabilizer. Human albumin solution is a commonly used colloid volume expander. *Also see colloid osmotic pressure.*

Aldosterone   The principal corticosteroid (mineralocorticoid) hormone released by the adrenal cortex. It is involved in the regulation of arterial blood pressure and extracellular fluid volume. It induces the reabsorption of sodium and water along with the excretion of potassium in renal distal convoluted tubules. Also, has an effect on sweat glands and salivary glands.

Alert

State of being watchful or ready.

Alexia

Inability to read. *Also see dyslexia.*

Alkalosis

A state in which the pH is elevated above 7.45. In primary *metabolic alkalosis*, the arterial CO_2 changes in the same direction as the pH ($\uparrow$ pH and $\uparrow$ $PaCO_2$). In primary *respiratory alkalosis*, the $PaCO_2$ and pH change in opposite directions ($\uparrow$ pH and $\downarrow$ $PaCO_2$). *Also see, pH, acidosis, buffer, and Henderson-Hasselbalch equation.*

Allergen

An agent (antigen) that evokes an allergic or inappropriate immune response. Common examples include: dust, pollen, animal fur, certain medications and latex.

Allergy

A state of hypersensitivity of the body's immune system caused by exposure to specific allergens. It is presumed to be mediated by histamine. A severe allergic response can result in anaphylactic shock.

All-Or-None Law

The statement that a given response will be produced to its maximum extent only in response to any stimulus equal to or greater than a threshold value. Action potentials obey the all-or-none law. *Also see action potential.*

Allosteric (site)

A site on an enzyme or protein that modulates the activity or efficiency of the enzyme or protein when occupied by certain molecules. It is distinct from the active or catalytic site of the enzyme or protein.

Alpha Motor neuron

Somatic motor neuron which innervates extrafusal skeletal muscle fibers. Stimulation results in an action potential in the innervated muscle and subsequent contraction.

Alpha Rhythm

Normal awake EEG waves that occur at a frequency of 8-12 hertz. It is also called alpha wave. *Also see electroencephalogram.*

Aminostatic Theory

See Food Intake.

Amnesia

Lack of memory about events occurring during a particular period of time. *Also see anterograde amnesia.*

Amniocentesis

A procedure that involves obtaining amniotic fluid through a trans-abdominal approach. Used in obstetrics to obtain information on fetal development and genetic composition.

Amnion

The inner of two fetal membranes surrounding the fetus during pregnancy; it contains amniotic fluid and is commonly termed the *"bag of waters."*

Amniotic Fluid

The fluid found within the amniotic cavity.

Amphoterism

The ability of a compound to behave both as an acid and as a base. Water and the bicarbonate ion are two prime examples. *From the Greek word "amphoteros," meaning "pertaining to both."*

Anabolic Steroids

Synthetic derivatives of testosterone, the naturally-occurring male anabolic hormone; they enhance protein synthesis.

Anabolism

Constructive metabolic process involving the input of energy (ATP); large organic molecules are produced from smaller precursor molecules.

Anaerobic respiration

The type of cellular respiration in which the final electron acceptor is an inorganic molecule other than oxygen. Far less ATP is produced compared to aerobic respiration.

Anaerobic Threshold

The level of exertion at which the body switches from aerobic to anaerobic metabolism; it is the point, during exercise, at which muscle oxygen demand outstrips the supply.

Anaphylaxis

A severe type I hypersensitivity reaction resulting from an antigen-antibody reaction on mast cells and subsequent mast cell degranulation. Release of histamine and other vasoactive substances occurs and in severe cases, total cardiovascular collapse may occur. Anaphylactoid reactions are clinically similar, but do not usually involve antigen-antibody interactions. Direct or complement activated release of vasoactive chemicals occurs. Latex allergy is an important cause of an anaphylactic reaction. *Also see hypersensitivity.*

Androgen

A male sex steroid hormone e.g. testosterone; produced primarily by the testes and to a lesser extent by the adrenal cortex. It controls development and maintenance of male characteristics.

Anemia

A reduction in circulating red blood cell mass or reduced hemoglobin concentration in blood; it results in diminished oxygen delivery to tissues and organs.

Anemia is usually detected by performing a complete blood cell count (primarily, Red Blood Cell count, Hematocrit and hemoglobin concentration).

The most common types of anemia are as follows:

Iron deficiency anemia - caused by (a) inadequate iron intake (b) chronic blood loss (c) impaired dietary iron absorption (d) pregnancy or lactation. Treatment is usually by dietary iron supplementation.

Aplastic anemia - Caused by destruction of the bone marrow by factors such as industrial chemical agents, radiation exposure or other physical factors, certain drugs and infections. It may also be congenital (Fanconi's anemia). In many cases, the cause is unknown.

Hemorrhagic anemia – Caused by excessive blood loss. Rapid (short-term) hemorrhage results in low RBC concentration, with compensation occurring in 3-6 weeks. Chronic hemorrhage is associated with impaired iron absorption and consequently, reduced hemoglobin, causing microcytic, hypochromic anemia. Treatment includes the following: (a) Arrest of bleeding (b) restoring blood volume with fluids and transfusion, and (c) Iron supplementation.

Sickle cell anemia – Caused by the presence of an abnormal type of hemoglobin (hemoglobin S) in red blood cells. These cells are prone to rapid hemolysis.

Megaloblastic anemia – Results from vitamin B12 and folic acid deficiency. Common causes include the following: (a) impaired intrinsic factor production – *pernicious anemia* (b) intestinal malabsorption (c) nutritional defects and (d) chronic liver disease.

Hemolytic anemia – Caused by excessive hemolysis of RBCs usually from hereditary causes. Common causes are spherocytosis, G6PD deficiency, certain drugs, Paroxysmal nocturnal hematuria and ABO or Rhesus incompatibility. *Also see sickle cell anemia.*

Aneurysm

A balloon-like deformity in the wall of a blood vessel or the heart. The wall weakens as the balloon enlarges and may eventually rupture resulting in life-threatening hemorrhage.

Angina Pectoris

A common symptom of myocardial ischemia. The angina pain is commonly referred to the left shoulder, arms and neck and may be accompanied by sweating, nausea and dizziness. It occurs when myocardial oxygen demand exceeds supply, e.g. excessive exercise in at risk persons, excitement and coronary artery disease (CAD). Severe cases result in myocardial death (infarction). *Also see Isosorbide dinitrate.*

Angiogenesis

The process by which new blood vessels are formed. Cancer cells utilize this process to grow and spread and anti-angiogenesis agents are being evaluated for treatment of human cancer. *Also see endothelial cell growth factor.*

Angiotensin II

A powerful vasoconstrictor; it is an eight-amino-acid polypeptide produced in the lungs by conversion from Angiotensin I (a ten-amino-acid precursor).

Angiotensin II elicits the following functions:

- Stimulates secretion of aldosterone by the adrenal cortex.
- Causes vasoconstriction via AT1 receptors
- Stimulates the adrenal cortex to release aldosterone, and thus, Na^+ and fluid retention
- Stimulates brain thirst centers
- Facilitates adrenergic function by enhanced sympathetic neuronal release and inhibition of noradrenaline re-uptake
- Stimulates secretion of ADH from the posterior pituitary; this increases renal fluid retention.

Angiotensin receptor blockers (ARBs) such as Valsartan are commonly used anti-hypertensives. Also, ACEI (Angiotensin converting enzyme inhibitors) are widely used in the treatment of hypertension and heart failure.

Angiotensin Converting Enzyme (ACE)

The enzyme that converts the inactive Angiotensin I to the active form (Angiotensin II). *Also see Angiotensin II and Bradykinin.*

Anion

A negatively charged ion e.g. chloride, thiocyanate or bicarbonate.

Anomia

Inability to recall the names of objects. Persons with this problem often can speak fluently but have to use other words to describe familiar objects.

Anosmia

Loss of the sense of smell.

Anterior

At or toward the front of an organism, organ, or part; the ventral surface.

Anterior Pituitary

See adenohypophysis.

Anterograde amnesia

Inability to consolidate information about ongoing events. Difficulty with new learning.

Antibody

An immunoglobulin molecule secreted by B-lymphocytes. Antibodies confer humoral immunity. Antibodies are present in the body or are produced in response to antigenic stimulation

Anticoagulant

An agent that inhibits blood clotting.

Anticoagulation

The process by which normal blood clotting is slowed thus preventing clot formation. Commonly referred to as "blood thinning." Used in the prevention and treatment of deep vein thrombosis (DVT), CAD, and during certain cardiovascular procedures. Commonly used anticoagulants include: Coumarin, Heparin, and Lovenox. *Also see warfarin.*

Anticodon

A triplet of nucleotide bases that constitutes the specific code within a loop of transfer RNA; allows recognition of a specific codon. The codon-anticodon matching is necessary for translation of the genetic code into a specific amino acid sequence. *Also see codon.*

Anticonvulsant

Medication used for the treatment of seizure disorder. Examples include: phenytoin, phenobarbitol, mysoline, tegretol, valproic acid, levetiracetam, and lamotrigine.

Antidepressant

Medications used for the treatment of depression.

Antidiuretic hormone (ADH)

A peptide hormone containing 9 amino acids; also known as *vasopressin*. It is secreted by the posterior pituitary gland. *ADH acts on the renal collecting ducts to stimulate water reabsorption.* It also constricts blood vessels, increases blood pressure, increases gastrointestinal motility and reduces urine excretion. Impairment of ADH secretion results in excessive loss of dilute urine, a condition known as diabetes insipidus (DI). There are two types of DI: central or nephrogenic. SIADH (syndrome of Inappropriate ADH) secretion occurs in the presence of different disease processes. It results in production of hypertonic urine in the presence of hyponatremia and decreased plasma osmolality. ADH is useful only in the treatment of central DI and is ineffective for nephrogenic DI. Various analogues of vasopressin are used in other areas such as: control of bleeding, esophageal varices, testing the concentrating ability of the kidneys, treatment of von Willebrand's disease, and in cardiopulmonary resuscitation.

Antigen

A molecule that stimulates the production of antibodies. *Also see Allergy and antibody.*

Antigenic Determinant Site

The location on the antigen molecule at which specific interaction occurs with particular antibodies.

Antiport

The counter-transport (or co-transport) of two molecules across a membrane in opposite directions. *Also see electrogenic Na⁺ pump.*

Antiserum

Serum which contains antibodies; it confers passive immunity.

Aorta

Largest systemic artery – receives blood from the left ventricle.

Aortic Bodies

Sensory receptors located in the aortic arch. They respond to changes in oxygen and carbon dioxide contents as well as blood pH.

Aortic Valve

One of the semilunar valves located between the left ventricle and the aorta; it opens during ventricular systole.

Apallic Syndrome

The behavior that accompanies diffuse bilateral degeneration of the cerebral cortex that sometimes follows anoxic brain injury. It describes patients with absent cortical function but with relatively intact brain stem function. Apallic syndrome is an older, non-specific term which has largely been replaced by persistent vegetative state.

Apathy

A lack of interest or concern.

Apex Beat

The point, on the precordium, of maximum cardiac pulsation.

Aphasia

Loss of the ability to express one's self and/or to understand language. Caused by damage to brain cells (involving Broca's area, the arcuate fasciculus, Wernicke's area, or the angular gyrus) rather than deficits in speech or hearing organs. Usually due to thromboembolism of a cerebral blood vessel. The various forms of aphasia are:

- *Expressive Aphasia:* Inability to find or formulate the words to express oneself despite knowing what one wants to say.
- *Fluent Aphasia:* Characterized by spontaneous use of language at normal speed that conveys little meaning.
- *Non-fluent Aphasia:* Characterized by awkward articulation, limited vocabulary, hesitant, slow speech output, restricted use of grammatical forms and a relative preservation of auditory comprehension.
- *Receptive Aphasia:* Problems in understanding what others attempt to communicate.
- *Subclinical Aphasia:* Refers to evidence of impaired linguistic processing on testing, which is not obvious in casual interactions.
- *Global Aphasia:* Severely limited residual ability to communicate with others. Includes both expressive and receptive aphasia.

Aphemia

The isolated loss of the ability to articulate words without loss of the ability to write or comprehend spoken language. *Also see apraxia.*

Apnea

The transient cessation of breathing. Types include central, obstructive and mixed. Central apnea is common in premature infants and obstructive sleep apnea (OSA) is a common feature of morbid obesity and tonsillar hypertrophy. *Also see obstructive sleep apnea.*

Apneustic Center

Center located in the lower part of the pons; in combination with the pneumotaxic center, controls the intensity and rate of respiration. *Also see pneumotaxic center.*

Apocrine Sweat Glands

Large skin glands that originate from the epidermis; they open into hair follicles and are innervated by sympathetic adrenergic nerve fibers.

Appetite

Craving or desire for a particular type of food.

Apraxia

Inability to carry out complex or skilled movements; not due to paralysis, sensory changes, or deficiencies in understanding. Two main forms exist:

Constructional Apraxia: Inability to assemble, build, draw, or copy accurately; not due to apraxia of single movements.

Ideomotor Apraxia: Deficit in the execution of a movement due to inability to access the instructions to muscles stored by prior motor experience.

Apoptosis

"Programmed cell death." It is the intrinsic physiological response of a cell to genotoxic cellular stressors (e.g. viral infection, physical or chemical damage or UV-light), thereby protecting the whole organism. There are three different mechanisms of apoptosis:

- Intrinsic or internal signal pathway arising from within the cell.
- Apoptosis induced by reactive oxygen species.
- Apoptosis triggered by activators (e.g. TNF-α and lymphotoxin) that bind to receptors on the cell surface.

Aquaporins

Membrane water channels found in many animal species. While being completely impermeable to protons, aquaporins enhance transmembrane transport of water and other small molecules.

Aqueous Humor

A transparent fluid between the cornea and the lens; it is produced by the ciliary body and provides nourishment for the cornea and the lens. *Also see vitreous humor.*

Arachnoid Villi

Microscopic projections of pia-arachnoid mater that extend into veins and venous sinuses of the dura.

Arousal

Being awake. Primitive state of alertness managed by the reticular activating system (extending from the medulla to the thalamus in the core of the brain stem) activating the cortex. Some degree of arousal is required for cognition to occur.

Artemisinin

A drug produced from the shrub *Artemisia Annua*; it is used for the treatment of multi-drug resistant falciparum malaria.

Arterial Pressure

See Blood Pressure.

Arterioles

Smallest branches of arteries; they have an average diameter of about 450 micrometer down to about 100 micrometer. Arterioles are the major determinant of vascular resistance because of their muscular walls.

Arteriosclerosis

An arterial disease associated with hardening and loss of elasticity of the vessel wall and luminal narrowing. Atherosclerosis is a form of arteriosclerosis characterized by deposition of cholesterol plaques (atheromas) in the vessel wall. Arteriosclerosis is a major cause of coronary artery and cerebrovascular diseases.

Arterio-venous Anastomoses

Structures which directly connect arterioles and veins thus bypassing the capillary bed. They are particularly important in the regulation of cutaneous blood flow and body temperature. Arterio-venous malformations (AVM) occur when large connections occur and may result in significant cardiovascular compromise.

Artery

A vessel that carries blood away from the heart.

Articulation

Movement of the lips, tongue, teeth and palate into specific patterns for purposes of speech. Also, a movable joint.

Artificial Respiration

Any method of respiratory support used when the natural spontaneous breathing ceases or is inadequate. Commonly used in cardiopulmonary resuscitation (CPR), intensive care, and during anesthesia. Includes everything from mouth -to- mouth breathing to use of various airway devices including a face mask, non-invasive ventilation, supraglottic airway devices, and endotracheal intubation.

Ascites

Accumulation of large amounts of fluid and protein in the peritoneal cavity. A common feature of liver disease and congestive heart failure. *Also see edema.*

Ascorbic Acid

A water-soluble organic acid; the L-enantiomer is commonly called Vitamin C. It functions as an antioxidant in biological systems. Dietary sources include oranges, strawberries, green peppers, green leafy vegetables, tomatoes, and raw cabbage.

Asphyxia

A pathological condition caused by a lack of oxygen to the tissues.

Aspiration

Inhalation of fluid, food or any foreign body into the lungs. Can cause a lung infection (pneumonia), or acute lung injury.

Associated Reaction

A non-purposeful movement that accompanies another movement (e.g., patient's arm may bend involuntarily when the patient yawns).

Association Areas

Parts of the cerebral cortex that receive and process signals from multiple regions of the motor and sensory cortex simultaneously. Also receives signals from subcortical structures.

Astereognosis

Inability to recognize objects by touch.

Asthma

A chronic inflammatory condition of the airways characterized by episodic, reversible bronchospasm, airway edema and mucus plugging. Associated with shortness of breath, wheezing, and exercise intolerance. Asthma is an important cause of morbidity and mortality. Treatment is with the use of bronchodilators, steroids, and newer specific medications. *Also see leukotrienes.*

Astigmatism

A visual error of refraction caused by a larger than normal curvature of the cornea in one of its planes. Correction is with a cylindrical lens. *Also see myopia and hyperopia.*

Astrocytes

Subtypes of neuroglial cells in the brain. They exist in two forms: fibrous astrocytes, predominant in bundles of myelinated nerve fibers and white mater of the brain and protoplasmic astrocytes, which are less fibrous and abundant in the grey mater around nerve cell bodies, dendrites, and synapses. *Also see glial cells.*

Ataxia

Uncoordinated movement of the limbs or trunk, usually due to cerebellar dysfunction.

Athetosis

Slow and confluent spontaneous movements arising commonly from lesions in the caudate nucleus, putamen, and sometimes in the ventrolateral nucleus of the thalamus.

Atopic Dermatitis

A chronic itchy skin irritation usually due to a general systemic allergic reaction; it is common in individuals with allergic conditions, e.g. asthma and hay fever.

ATPase (Adenosine Triphosphatase)

The enzyme involved in the maintenance of the concentration gradients for Na^+ and K^+ ions across the cell membrane. By inhibiting this enzyme, cardiac glycosides like digoxin produce an increase in intracellular Na^+ and Ca^{2+} ions and a positive inotropic effect.

Atresia

Denotes absence of an opening; e.g. absence of a segment of the intestines or the esophagus in a newborn.

Atrial Fibrillation

A form of abnormal heart rhythm in which there is an uncoordinated, repetitive excitation of the atrial wall with loss of normal atrio-ventricular synchrony. Peripheral pulses are 'irregularly irregular'. Condition is common in the elderly and associated with a sedentary lifestyle. It is an important cause of strokes and peripheral thromboembolism arising from the heart. The primary goal of treatment is control of ventricular rate.

Atrioventricular Node (A-V Node)

One of the impulse-conducting, auto rhythmic fibers in the heart; it is a small mass of cells and connective tissue located in the lower, posterior region of the atrial septum. It transmits impulses received from the sino-atrial node (SAN) to the ventricular walls. *Also see Cardiac Conduction System.*

Atrioventricular Valve (A-V Valves)

Situated between the atria and ventricles. There are two types: tricuspid and mitral valves. The valves allow uni-directional blood flow from the atria to the ventricles and prevent backflow into the atria.

Atrial Natriuretic Factor

A vasodilator peptide secreted by the atria in response to increased atrial volume and pressure; it stimulates urinary excretion of sodium. *Also see Natriuretic hormone.*

Atria

The upper receiving chambers of the heart; located above their respective ventricles.

Atrophy

A wasting away or decrease in size of part of the body caused by a lack of nourishment, inactivity or denervation. Muscle wasting from nerve damage is an example.

Atropine

An alkaloid drug, derived from the Belladonna plant (Atropa Belladona). It is an anticholinergic that antagonizes the action of acetylcholine at muscarinic receptor sites and is used clinically to treat or prevent bradycardia (slow heart rate), dry secretions (antisialologue), as an antispasmodic, and to dilate the pupils. It is also used to block the muscarinic effects of anticholinesterases like neostigmine in anesthetic practice. Related drugs include glycopyrrolate and scopolamine (hyoscine). *Also see acetylcholine.*

Attendant care

Provision of assistance in activities of daily living for individuals with some form of disability.

Audiologist

A specialist that evaluates hearing defects and assists in the rehabilitation of such patients.

Audiometry

Assessment of hearing ability. It determines an individual's hearing levels and the ability to discriminate between different sound intensities. *Also see Rinne's and Weber tests and deafness.*

Auerbach's Plexus

Intrinsic nerve plexus located between the outer longitudinal and inner circular smooth muscle layers of the gut wall. Also called myenteric plexus.

Auscultatory Blood Pressure Measurement

An indirect method of blood pressure measurement; involves the use of a stethoscope placed usually over the brachial artery and inflating a cuff placed around the arm. Gradual cuff deflation while listening for *Korotkoff sounds* allows measurement of systolic and diastolic pressures. *Also see blood pressure.*

Autoantibody

An antibody that acts against (and is formed in response to) tissues of the organism that produces it. Believed to be the basis for certain autoimmune diseases.

Autocrine Regulation

A type of regulation in which a cell releases substances that regulate the function of the same cell by binding to receptors on the cell surface. Prostaglandins are examples of autocrine regulators.

Autonomic Nervous System (ANS)

An involuntary neural system responsible for rapid control of visceral organs functions and homeostasis. Autonomic neurons have two components: *preganglionic* and *postganglionic.* The ANS controls activity of visceral organs e.g. heart and smooth muscles; it is responsible for the control of blood pressure, heart rate, breathing, body temperature, and stress response. Axons of preganglionic fibers originate in the central nervous system (CNS) and synapse with cell bodies of postganglionic fibers at autonomic ganglia outside the CNS. The two main subdivisions of the ANS are: *sympathetic* and *parasympathetic.* These two divisions act in an antagonistic manner on visceral organs (when one stimulates, the other inhibits). *Also see parasympathetic and sympathetic nervous systems.*

Autonomic Receptors

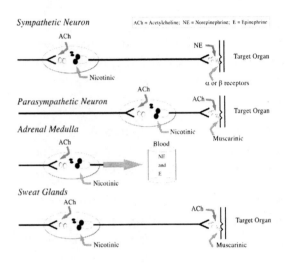

Receptors of the parasympathetic (cholinergic) and sympathetic (adrenergic) nervous system. There are two subtypes of cholinergic receptors: nicotinic and muscarinic. *Nicotinic receptors* are located on motor endplate of skeletal muscles, at autonomic neuronal synapses and on the chromaffin cells of the adrenal medulla. Acetylcholine, nicotine and carbachol are specific agonists at nicotinic receptor sites. Nicotinic receptors are blocked by ganglion-blocking drugs e.g. curare and hexamethonium; however, hexamethonium does not block nicotinic receptors on motor endplate membranes. Muscarinic receptors are located on target organs of the parasympathetic nervous system e.g. gastrointestinal tract (GIT), bladder, heart, genitalia and bronchioles. Muscarinic receptors are also found in target organs innervated by postganglionic cholinergic neurons of sympathetic nerves. Muscarinic receptors are stimulated by acetylcholine and antagonized by atropine. *Also see adrenergic receptors, cholinergic receptors, and acetylcholine.*

Autoregulation

The intrinsic phenomenon by which blood flow to an organ, especially vital organs, remains constant despite changes in perfusion pressure. Autoregulation is achieved by metabolic and myogenic mechanisms and is independent of extrinsic (neural or humoral) control. The cerebral circulation exhibits classic autoregulation that maintains cerebral blood flow (CBF) within a range of mean arterial pressures (MAP). Outside of these limits (50-150mmHg), CBF varies directly with MAP.

Autosomal Dominant (gene)

A single abnormal gene located on one of the autosomal chromosomes and inherited from one parent. There is a 50% chance to pass from parent to child. Examples: Achondroplasia (dwarfism), Osteogenesis Imperfecta, and Huntington's disease.

Axon

The long process of a nerve cell that conducts impulses away from the cell body of the neuron.

Axonal Transport

The transport of materials through the axon of a neuron. This usually occurs from the cell body to the end of the axon, but retrograde (backward) transport can also occur.

Azotemia

Elevated blood levels of urea or other nitrogen-containing compounds. Also called *Uremia*. It is present in advanced renal impairment and severe dehydration. *Also see renal failure.*

B

Babinski sign

Dorsiflexion of the big toe and fanning out of the other toes when the sole of the foot is stroked. It is usually an indication of upper motor neuron dysfunction.

Bacteria

A group of single cell prokaryotic microorganisms which exist in either free-living forms or as parasites. Some bacteria have physiologic functions but a majority are pathogenic (cause disease).

Bacteriophage

A virus that infects and lyses bacteria.

Bag Fibers (nuclear)

See nuclear bag fibers.

Bainbridge Reflex

An atrial reflex elicited by stretch receptors in the atria; it is mediated by afferent vagal signals to the medulla and efferent vagal and sympathetic signals. Results in increased heart rate and force of contraction.

Ball-And-Socket Joint

A freely-movable type of joint in which the articular surface presents a ball-like shape which fits into a cavity. The hip and shoulder joints are examples.

Ballism

Dysfunction of the basal ganglia associated with violent, flailing movements of the limbs (ballistic movements).

Baroreceptors

Pressure receptors located in the walls of the atria, aortic arch, carotid sinuses, and vena cava.

Barr body

A dark-staining microscopic structure found in the nuclei of females; it contains an inactive X chromosome. Also called *sex chromatin. Also see chromatin.*

Basal Body

A cylindrical structure present in the cell cytoplasm and located at the base of a cilium or a flagellum.

Basal Ganglia

Large clusters of nerve cells or gray matter deep within the cerebral hemispheres, the upper brain stem, the striatum, and the substantia nigra. Its main function is on the motor cortex where it modulates movement. Disorders of movement such as Parkinson's disease and Huntington's disease are caused by disturbances in the basal ganglia. *Also see Parkinson's disease and Ballism.*

Basal Metabolic Rate (BMR)

The minimum energy level required for performance of bodily functions; it is usually measured under basal conditions: (a) about 12 hours after the last meal (b) after a night of restful sleep (c) no exercise or physical activity at least 1 hour preceding the test (d) absence of emotional excitement (e) surrounding temperature must be comfortable (preferably, between 68° and 80°F). Average BMR value in a 70kg man is 65-70 calories per hour.

Basement Membrane

A structural layer that anchors epithelial tissue to underlying connective tissue.

Basilar Membrane

A fibrous membrane that supports the organ of Corti in the cochlea; it separates the scala media from the scala tympani.

Basophil

A type of white blood cells (leukocyte) with a characteristic two-lobed nucleus and bluish-black cytoplasmic granules. Basophils contain and are capable of releasing histamine and serotonin and constitute 0.5-3% of the total blood leukocytes.

B-Cell lymphocytes

The type of lymphocytes that undergo maturation in the bone marrow; they can be transformed by antigens into antibody-producing plasma cells. *Also see lymphocytes, plasma cells, and humoral immunity.*

Belching

A normal process for relieving gaseous distension of the stomach. Also called *eructation*.

Benign

Denotes a condition that is not malignant or life-threatening. Commonly used to define tumors.

Beta cells (ß-cells)

The insulin producing cells of the islet of Langerhans in the pancreas.

Beta Wave

Electroencephalogram (EEG) wave associated with the sleep-wake cycle, predominant in the awake, aroused state. Frequency is between 12 and 30 hertz. *Also see electroencephalogram.*

Bicuspid valve

A heart valve with two cusps. The mitral valve is a bicuspid valve located between the left atrium and left ventricle. A bicuspid aortic valve is abnormal.

Bile

Secretion produced by the liver and stored temporarily in the gallbladder; it contains bile salts, bile pigments, cholesterol, and other molecules. Bile is released into the small intestine where it emulsifies fats.

Bile Salts   Salts of bile acids e.g. glycocholate and taurocholate.

Bilirubin   A yellowish breakdown product of the heme portion of hemoglobin. It is present in plasma bound to albumin and is conjugated in the liver by glucoronic acid or sulfate. The accumulation of bilirubin in the body causes jaundice. The normal serum bilirubin is 0.5mg/dL. Jaundice occurs when the concentration rises to about three times normal. Jaundice is usually classified as hemolytic (unconjugated or indirect hyperbilirubinemia) or obstructive (conjugated or direct hyperbilirubinemia). Conversion of bilirubin to lumirubin (shorter half life) by white light is the basis for the use of phototherapy in the treatment of neonatal jaundice. *Also see jaundice and kernicterus.*

Biliverdin   The unstable breakdown product of heme that is rapidly converted to bilirubin.

Biotin   A water-soluble B-complex vitamin found in large amounts in certain foods such as green vegetables, nuts, milk and cereals. Biotin plays a role in carbon dioxide transfer and is therefore important for fat and carbohydrate metabolism. Hair loss and dermatitis are characteristic features of biotin deficiency.

Bipolar Cell   A neuronal cell type located in the retina; it relays signals from the rods, cones and horizontal cells to the plexiform layer.

Bitemporal Hemianopia   Blindness in both temporal visual fields. Tumors in the optic chiasm such as pituitary tumors, craniopharyngiomas, and suprasellar tumors are common causes.

Bladder (urinary)   A balloon-shaped muscular and distensible organ located inside the pelvis; it serves as a reservoir for urine. Emptying of the bladder is under the control of the micturition reflex, mediated via parasympathetic and sympathetic nerves.

Blastocyst   The stage of early pre-embryonic development. It consists of a cluster of cells called the inner cell mass, which forms the embryo, and an outer layer (trophoblast), which gives rise to the placenta and other supporting tissues necessary for fetal development.

Blastula

The fluid-filled hollow ball of cells formed prior to the formation of the gastrula during early embryonic development in mammals.

Blind Spot

Area of the eye where the optic nerve passes through the retina. It is devoid of rods and cones, hence the name.

Blood

A type of connective tissue in which cells are separated by plasma.

Blood-Brain Barrier

A system of specialized capillary endothelial cells that selectively protects the central nervous system from circulating harmful substances whilst supplying the brain with required nutrients for proper function. The blood brain barrier involves both physical (tight junctions) and metabolic (enzymes) barriers and is of great importance in the selective permeation of medications into the brain.

Blood Pressure

Blood Pressure (BP) is a measure of the driving force for blood flow. Some factors that influence BP include: blood volume, vascular resistance, age, family history and diet. In simple physiologic terms, BP is represented mathematically as: $BP = CO \times TPR$, where

CO = cardiac output and TPR = total peripheral resistance. Blood pressure is usually measured indirectly by means of a sphygmomanometer. The systolic and diastolic pressures can be estimated by *palpation* or *auscultation*. Cannulation of a peripheral artery is used for continuous BP measurements, especially in the intensive care setting and during major surgical procedures. *Also see auscultatory blood pressure measurement and hypertension.*

Bohr Effect

Describes the principle that increased H^+ concentration resulting from increased CO_2 levels shifts the O_2-hemoglobin dissociation curve to the right (decreased affinity). This facilitates release (unloading) of oxygen from hemoglobin at the tissue level. *Also see Haldane effect and Oxyhemoglobin Dissociation Curve.*

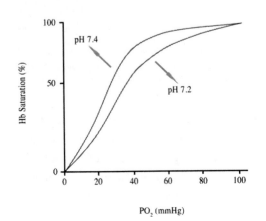

Bombesin
A tetradecapeptide compound extracted from the skin of some European frogs; it stimulates gastric acid secretion in mammals by releasing gastrin.

Bone
A type of connective tissue with a hard matrix and made up of mineral salts.

Bony Labyrinth
A system of bony tubes located in the vestibular apparatus of the inner ear; it has three parts: a central cavity (the vestibule), three semicircular canals (lateral, posterior and superior) and the cochlea (a snail-shaped spiral tube).

Bowman's Capsule (Glomerular Capsule)
The cup-like closed end of the nephron.

Bradycardia
A decreased heart rate (less than 60 beats/minute in adults).

Bradykinesia
A disease of the basal ganglia manifested by slowness in initiating movements.

Bradykinin
A nonapeptide kinin released from plasma kininogens. Produces vasodilatation and mediates pain. Bradykinin is inactivated by angiotensin converting enzyme (ACE), the same enzyme that converts angiotensin I to the active angiotensin II. ACE inhibitors can lead to accumulation of bradykinin and other kinins and this may explain the allergy-like symptoms, cough, and the rare but serious angioedema that may be seen with use of these drugs. *Also see Kallikrein, Angiotensin II, and Angiotensin Converting Enzyme.*

Brain
The part of the central nervous system located in the cranial cavity. Vertebrate brain has three components: hindbrain, midbrain and forebrain. It is responsible for coordination and control of body functions and memory storage.

Brain-Derived Neurotrophic Factor
A CNS protein that promotes survival of dorsal root ganglion neurons.

Brain Stem
Part of the brain consisting of the medulla oblongata, pons, and midbrain.

Broca's Area
Located in the posterior part of the inferior temporal gyrus of the left hemisphere; it is important in speech and language articulation.

Bronchedema

Fluid accumulation in and swelling of the bronchial mucosa.

Bronchiole

The smallest of the air passages in the lungs; terminates in the alveoli.

Brown Fat

A thermogenic type of adipose tissue most prominent in newborns and small infants. Mostly located between the shoulder blades and in the mediastinum. Used for temperature regulation in newborns since they lack a shivering mechanism.

Brush Border

Densely populated microvilli of intestinal epithelial cells.

Buffer

A molecule or system that resists changes in pH by reacting with a strong acid or base to form a weaker acid or base, respectively. In the body, buffer systems consist of a weak acid and its conjugate base. The carbonic acid-bicarbonate buffer system is the most important in the body. *Also see pH, acidosis and alkalosis.*

Bulb (Olfactory)

A cortical structure which contains the initial relay of neurons in the olfactory pathway.

Bulbourethral glands

Glands that secrete viscous fluid into the male urethra during sexual arousal; also called Cowper's glands.

Bulk Transport

A process by which materials are transported into a cell by phagocytosis or endocytosis and out of a cell by exocytosis.

Bundle of His

One of the specialized, rapidly-conducting, cardiac fibers that originate in the AV node and extend down the atrioventricular septum to the apex of the heart. Impulses from the bundle of His are transmitted to the left and right bundle branches and then into the Purkinje system. Disruption of this system results in varying degrees of heart block. *Also see Cardiac Conduction System.*

Bungarotoxin

Protein constituent of the venom of certain poisonous snakes; it combines irreversibly with acetylcholine at the neuromuscular junction.

Bursa

A fluid-filled sac-like structure that is lined by synovial membrane and near a joint; it facilitates movements across joints. Inflammation of the periarticular tissues causes *Bursitis.*

C

Cable Properties	Concepts that explain how nerves and muscles act as cables that conduct electrical activity.
Calcitonin (Thyrocalcitonin)	A polypeptide hormone produced by the C cells of the thyroid gland; it lowers blood calcium levels and acts as an antagonist of parathyroid hormone. *Also see parathyroid hormone.*
Calcitonin Gene-Related Peptide (cGRP)	A potent endogenous neuropeptide vasodilator found in large amounts in the brain, gut, and perivascular nerves. It also is associated with substance P in neurons.
Calcium	An important mineral responsible for healthy bones and teeth, nerve conduction, and muscle contraction. Also involved with blood clotting.
Calcium Channel Blockers	Drugs that inhibit the influx of calcium ions through membrane calcium channels. Examples include Verapamil, Diltiazem, Nifedipine, Nicardipine, and Nimodipine. They have wide clinical application especially in the treatment of cardiac tachyarrhythmias, hypertension, coronary artery disease, tocolysis (uterine relaxation), and prevention of cerebral vasospasm. *Also see L-type and T-type channels.*
Calmodulin	A calcium-dependent regulatory protein located within the cytoplasm of target cells. The calcium-calmodulin system is a mode for transduction of hormonal signals.
Calorie	The amount of heat required to raise the temperature of 1 gram of water by 1 $^{\circ}$C. It is the unit for heat energy.
Calsequestrin	A Ca^{2+}-binding protein located within the lumen of the terminal cisterns of the sarcoplasmic reticulum.
cAMP (Cyclic Adenosine Monophosphate)	ATP-related compound that acts as a second messenger in the action of many hormones including catecholamine, polypeptide, and glycoprotein hormones. It serves to mediate the effects of these hormones on their target cells. It is metabolized by phosphodiesterase enzyme (PDE). PDE inhibitors such as amrinone and milrinone are potent dilating inotropes used for circulatory support. Other non-specific PDEIs are methylxanthines (used for treating bronchoconstriction) and caffeine. *Also see phosphodiesterase.*

Canal Of Schlemm

Terminal outflow compartment for aqueous humor from the eye; it empties into extraocular veins.

Cancer

A malignant tumor characterized by uncontrolled cell growth and the ability to invade tissues and metastasize.

Capacitation

The post-ejaculatory processes that occur in spermatozoa; it renders them capable of fertilizing ova.

Capillaries

Microscopic blood vessels that connect arterioles to venules; permit exchanges of molecules between blood and tissue fluid.

Capsaicin

Active principle in pepper plant (capsicum). Selectively destroys certain sensory neurons and also depletes sensory nerves of substance P. Used in the treatment of certain types of pain.

Carbohydrate

An organic compound characterized by the presence of carbon, hydrogen, and oxygen in a ratio of 1:2:1. It includes monosaccharides, disaccharides, and polysaccharides.

Carbonic Anhydrase

An enzyme present in red blood cells that catalyzes the formation of carbonic acid from CO_2 and water and catalyzes its dissociation to hydrogen ions and bicarbonate. Besides CO_2 transport, it is also involved in aqueous humor formation. Acetazolamide (Diamox) is a carbonic anhydrase inhibitor that is used for the treatment of glaucoma.

Carboxyhemoglobin

An abnormal form of hemoglobin in which the heme is bound to carbon monoxide (CO). Because the affinity of CO for hemoglobin is about 250 times that of oxygen, oxygen transport is severely impaired. Smokers have a high level of carboxyhemoglobin and CO poisoning can occur from faulty heating systems, car exhausts, and burns. Treatment is with oxygen therapy. In severe cases, hyperbaric therapy may be required.

Carboxypeptidase

Pancreatic proteolytic enzyme secreted in the inactive form, procarboxypeptidase; it removes amino acids from the C-terminal ends of peptide chains.

Cardiac Conducting system

A system of highly specialized cardiac muscle fibers which transmit impulses from the pacemaker (SA

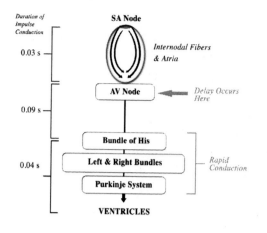

node) into the myocardium. Figure is a schematic representation of the conducting system of the heart showing the various fibers, relative conduction velocities and the duration of impulse conduction in the various fibers.

SA node: 60-80 beats/min

Atrioventricular (AV) node: (40-60 beats/min). Delay occurs here, to enable ventricular filling during diastole.

AV bundle (bundle of His): 40 beats/min

Purkinje fibers: Intrinsic rate = 15-20 beats/min

Cardiac Cycle

Contraction and relaxation of the heart associated with the heart beat; duration is 0.8 seconds.

Cardiac Muscle

Specialized, striated, involuntary muscle tissue found only in the heart.

Cardiac Output (CO)

The volume of blood pumped per minute by each ventricle. Mathematically, CO = Heart Rate (HR) x Stroke Volume (SV). It is about 5liters/min in an adult.

Cardiogenic Shock

Type of shock resulting from a primary cardiac etiology. Myocardial infarction (heart attack) is the most common cause. In cardiogenic shock, organ perfusion is severely impaired. Inotropes or other mechanical cardiac support are usually required and mortality rate is high. *Also see shock.*

Carotid Bodies

A cluster of baroreceptors, chemoreceptors and supporting cells located at the bifurcation of the common carotid artery. They detect changes in blood pressure, arterial blood gases (pO_2, pCO_2, pH), and temperature.

Carotid Sinus

Dilated portion of the vasculature at the bifurcation of the carotid arteries; it contains baroreceptors.

Carrier-Mediated Transport

Transport of molecules and ions requiring action of specific membrane protein carriers. May be subdivided into facilitated diffusion and active transport.

Catecholamines

Ethylamine derivatives of catechol; includes epinephrine, norepinephrine, dopamine and related compounds. Synthesis occurs in the axoplasm and in the secretory vesicles of adrenergic neurons. First, tyrosine is converted to DOPA (dihydroxyphenylalanine) by a hydroxylase enzyme; next, by decarboxylation, DOPA is converted into dopamine, which is transported into the vesicles. Dopamine is converted to norepinephrine by hydroxylation. In the adrenal medulla, 80% of the norepinephrine is converted into epinephrine by methylation. The released norepinephrine acts on postsynaptic receptors and is inactivated by (a) reuptake into the presynaptic neuron and (b) degradation by enzymes: monoamine oxidase (MAO) and Catechol-O-Methyl-Transferase (COMT). Natural catecholamines (epinephrine and dopamine) and synthetic catecholamines (isoproterenol and dobutamine) are widely used in clinical practice for various cardiovascular derangements. Epinephrine is the most important drug used during cardiopulmonary resuscitation. Ephedrine, metaraminol and phenylephrine are synthetic *non-catecholamines. Also see autonomic receptors, adrenergic receptors and parasympathetic nervous system.*

Caveolae

Sac-like invaginations of the cell membrane found mainly in smooth muscle. They are rudimentary analogues of the T-tubular system in skeletal muscles.

Cell-To-Cell Contacts

Specialized contacts between adjacent cardiac and smooth muscle cells that permit mechanical linkage and communication.

Cellular Respiration

Metabolic pathways that result in energy production in a cell.

Central Nervous System (CNS)

Part of the nervous system comprising the brain and the spinal cord. *Also see peripheral nervous system.*

Central Venous Pressure (CVP)

Pressure in the right atrium and the thoracic vena cavae; measured by central venous cannulation. It is a measure of right heart filling pressures and function. Left sided heart function is assessed by pulmonary artery catheterization. *Also see preload.*

Centriole

An organelle present in the cell; it forms the spindle apparatus during cell division.

Centromere

The central portion of a chromosome that provides attachment for the chromosomal arms.

Cerebellum

Part of the metencephalon of the brain that is posterior to the medulla oblongata and pons; it serves to coordinate skeletal muscle movements.

Cerebral Cortex

The thin, convoluted outer layer of gray matter covering the cerebral hemispheres; it is responsible for voluntary movement, sensation, and consciousness.

Cerebral Ischemia

Inadequate cerebral perfusion. Occurs when cerebral blood flow (CBF) falls below a critical level. Normal CBF is 50ml/100g/min.

Cerebral Palsy (CP)

CP is defined as a collection of central motor system disorders – spastic, choreathetotic, ataxic, dystonic or mixed, originating from a non-progressive neurological insult, sustained perinatally or in early childhood.

Cerebral Lateralization

Specialization of function of each cerebral hemisphere; e.g. language ability is lateralized to the left hemisphere in most people.

Cerebrospinal Fluid (CSF)

Fluid formed by the choroid plexus and located in the lateral, third, and fourth ventricles. Acts as a protective cushion for the brain and spinal cord. Sampling for diagnostic purposes is by a lumbar puncture.

Ceruloplasmin

A copper carrying plasma protein produced in the liver.

Chemical Senses

Senses of taste (gustation) and smell (olfaction).

Chemiosmotic Theory

The theory that oxidative phosphorylation within mitochondria is driven by the development of a H^+ gradient across the inner mitochondria membrane.

Chemoreceptors

Sensory receptors that are sensitive to chemical changes in blood and other body fluids; there are two types: peripheral and central chemoreceptors. Peripheral chemoreceptors are located in the carotid and aortic bodies; they detect changes in the blood pH, pO_2, and pCO_2. Central chemoreceptors are located in the medulla and are sensitive mainly to changes in pCO_2, pH and to a lesser extent, changes in pO_2.

Chemotaxis

The directional movement of cells towards chemical substances as occurs with leukocytes.

Chenodeoxycholic Acid

A product of cholesterol breakdown; combines with glycine or taurine to form conjugated bile acids.

Chewing

Mechanical grinding of food in the mouth; breaks down the food particles into smaller bits for the action of salivary juice. Also called mastication.

Cheyne-Stokes Respiration

Abnormal breathing pattern in which tidal volume waxes and wanes cyclically with recurrent periods of apnea. Seen in congestive heart failure and certain central nervous disorders.

Chief Cells

Also called peptic cells; present in gastric glands and responsible for pepsinogen secretion.

Chloride Shift

The diffusion of chloride into red blood cells as HCO_3^- diffuses out of the cell. This occurs in tissue capillaries as a result of the production of carbonic acid from carbon dioxide. Serves to maintain electrical neutrality in the cell.

Cholecystokinin (CCK)

A hormone secreted by the duodenal mucosa; it stimulates contraction of the gallbladder and enhances secretion of pancreatic juice.

Cholesterol

Present in diet and absorbed from the gastrointestinal tract. It also is produced endogenously in cells. It serves as a precursor for steroid hormones produced by the gonads and adrenal cortex. *Also see lipoproteins.*

Cholinergic Receptors

Receptors of the parasympathetic nervous system. There are two types: nicotinic and muscarinic. Nicotinic receptors are located on the motor endplate of skeletal muscles, on autonomic neuronal synapses, and on the chromaffin cells of the adrenal medulla. Acetylcholine, nicotine, and carbachol are specific agonists at nicotinic receptors. Nicotinic receptors are blocked by ganglion-blocking drugs e.g. curare and hexamethonium and non-depolarizing muscle relaxants like pancuronium, rocuronium, and vecuronium. Hexamethonium however does not block nicotinic receptors on motor endplate membranes. Muscarinic receptors are located on effector organs of the parasympathetic nervous system e.g. heart, bronchioles, gastrointestinal tract (GIT), bladder, and genitalia. They are also found in effector organs innervated by postganglionic cholinergic neurons of sympathetic nerves. Muscarinic receptors are stimulated by Acetylcholine and antagonized by atropine. *Also see acetylcholine and atropine.*

Cholinesterase

See acetylcholinesterase.

Chondrocyte   A cartilage forming cell.

Chordae Tendinae   Fine filaments located on the edges of the atrioventricular valves; they prevent eversion of the valves during ventricular systole.

Chorea   A spectrum of central nervous system disorders (usually of the basal ganglia) characterized by rapid, flicking, and purposeless movements of facial and extremity muscles.

Choroid Plexus   Site of cerebrospinal fluid (CSF) formation. *Also see CSF.*

Christmas Factor   Clotting factor IX; synthesized by hepatocytes.

Chromatids   Duplicated chromosomes that are joined together at the centromere; they separate during cell division.

Chromosome   Rod-like structure in the nucleus that contains DNA and associated proteins. Also contains RNA that is made according to the genetic instructions in the DNA. Chromosomes are in a compact form during cell division hence, they become visible as discrete structures under light microscopy at this time.

Chylomicrons   Small particles of triglycerides, phospholipids, and cholesterol combined with proteins in intestinal epithelial cells. They are secreted into lymphatic capillaries of intestinal villi.

Chyme   A semi-fluid mixture of partially digested food and digestive juice that passes from the stomach into the small intestine.

Chymosin   *See Rennin.*

Chymotrypsin   A pancreatic proteolytic enzyme.

Cilia   Minute hair-like structures which extend from the cell surface; they beat in a coordinated fashion and are used for cell motility.

Cimetidine   A histamine (H_2) receptor antagonist. Used as an antacid in clinical practice. Other H_2 antagonists are ranitidine and famotidine.

Circadian Rhythms   Regular physiological or behavioral changes that repeat at about every 24 hours.

Cirrhosis

Chronic liver disease characterized by replacement of liver tissue with inactive fibrous scar tissue; commonly caused by excessive alcohol consumption and hepatitis. *Also see portal system.*

Clonal Selection Theory

States that active immunity is produced by the development of clones of lymphocytes that are able to respond to a particular antigen.

Clone

A group of cells derived from a single parent cell by asexual reproduction. All the cells have an identical genetic constitution.

Clotting factors

Factors involved in the coagulation process.

See table:

Factors	Common Names
Factor I	Fibrinogen
Factor II	Prothrombin
Factor III	tissue thromboplastin (tissue factor)
Factor IV	ionized calcium (Ca^{2+})
Factor V	labile factor or proaccelerin
Factor VII	stable factor or proconvertin
Factor VIII	antihemophilic factor
Factor IX	plasma thromboplastin component, Christmas factor
Factor X	Stuart-Prower factor
Factor XI	plasma thromboplastin antecedent
Factor XII	Hageman factor
Factor XIII	fibrin-stabilizing factor

Coagulation

The hemostatic process by which solid fibrin clots are formed; clot formation arrests bleeding and facilitates the repair of damaged blood vessels.

Cobalamins

Porphyrin-like ring structures with a centrally placed cobalt atom. *Also see cyanocobalamin.*

Cochlea

Part of the inner ear; it contains the spiral organ (Organ of Corti), which is responsible for hearing. *Also see Organ of Corti.*

Codon

The "triplet" nucleotide bases in mRNA that controls the amino acid sequence in a protein molecule synthesized by a cell. *Also see anticodon.*

Coenzyme

A non-protein organic molecule that combines with and activates specific enzyme proteins.

Cofactors

Usually inorganic ions like Ca^{2+}, Mg^{2+}, selenium; they are required for the catalytic action of an enzyme.

Colipase

A protein that prevents the inactivation of pancreatic lipase by bile salts.

Collecting Duct

Tubular structure within the kidney that transports urine through the renal medulla to the renal pelvis; water is reabsorbed here under the influence of ADH hence urine in the collecting duct is hypertonic to plasma. In nephrogenic diabetes insipidus, there is a loss of response to ADH.

Color Blindness

Inability to distinguish between some colors; it is due to a congenital absence of one or more types of cones.

Complement

A system of over 30 different plasma proteins that provide nonspecific defense against microbes.

Conducting Zone

Consists of the trachea, bronchi, up to the terminal bronchioles; part of the respiratory system responsible for the transmission of air to the gas-exchanging areas of the lungs. Does not participate in gas exchange. These areas constitute the anatomic dead space. *Also see dead space and respiratory zone.*

Cones

Sensory receptors in the retina that detect color and provide a high visual acuity.

Congestive heart failure (CHF)

Inability of the heart to maintain an adequate output to meet the body's metabolic needs. The most common causes are hypertension and coronary artery disease. Impaired venous return can cause peripheral edema and ascites.

Conjunctivitis

Inflammation of the conjunctiva; sometimes called "pink eye."

Connective Tissue

Type of tissue characterized by an abundance of cells separated by fiber-rich matrix.

Consensual Light Reflex

See Pupillary light reflex.

Contralateral

Originating or occurring in a corresponding part on the opposite side of the body.

Cornea

The transparent anterior structure forming the outer layer of the eyeball.

Corpora Quadrigemina

Part of the midbrain (mesencephalon) consisting of the superior (for visual reflexes) and inferior (for auditory reflexes) colliculi.

Corpus Callosum

The major nerve fiber tract that connects the two cerebral hemispheres. Agenesis of the corpus callosum is a rare congenital anomaly.

Cortex (cerebral)

See Cerebral Cortex.

Corticospinal Tract

Also called pyramidal tracts. A type of descending fiber tracts from the cerebral cortex to the anterior motor neurons in the spinal cord. Most of the corticospinal tracts fibers decussate (cross-over) in the medulla and give rise to the lateral corticospinal tracts. The uncrossed fibers form the anterior corticospinal tracts. Together with the extra pyramidal tracts, it controls motor activity. Lesions result in upper motor neuron lesion. *Also see upper motor neuron and motor neuron disease.*

Corticotropin-Releasing Hormone (CRH)

A 41 amino acid peptide originating in cells of the paraventricular nucleus of the hypothalamus; stimulates the release of adrenocorticotropic hormone (ACTH).

Cortisol

See corticosteroids.

Corticosteroids

Steroid hormones of the adrenal cortex; comprises glucocorticoids (e.g. cortisol and corticosterone) and mineralocorticoids (e.g. aldosterone).

Cotransport

Also called secondary active transport or coupled transport. Membrane transport in which energy required for *uphill* movement of a molecule is obtained from the *downhill* transport of Na$^+$ into the cell. ATP energy is required indirectly.

Countercurrent Multiplier System

Interaction occurring between the descending and ascending limbs of the loop of Henle in the kidney; it results in the multiplication of the solute concentration in the interstitial fluid of the renal medulla.

Creatine Phosphate (Phosphocreatine)

Organic phosphate molecule in muscle cell containing high-energy phosphate bond required for ATP synthesis.

Creatinine
Nitrogenous end product of creatine phosphate metabolism; it is excreted by the kidneys.

Crenation
The shrinking of red blood cells in a hypertonic solution as a result of osmosis; the RBCs acquire a notched or scalloped appearance.

Cretinism
A condition caused by impaired development of the thyroid in an infant; it can result in stunted growth and mental retardation.

Crossed Extensor Reflex
An integrated contralateral reflex action in which flexion on one side is accompanied by inhibition of the flexors and facilitation of the extensors on the opposite limb.

Crypts of Lieberkühn
Invaginations of the small intestinal epithelium into the submucosa; they contain specialized secretory cells.

Cryptorchidism (Undescended Testis)
Failure of the testes to descend into the scrotum and instead remain in the body cavity, most commonly in the spermatic canal. Surgical treatment is often required.

Curare
A neuromuscular blocking drug first used as an arrow poison by native South Americans. Acts by competitive blockade of acetylcholine at the neuromuscular junction. It has largely been replaced by newer agents but remains an interesting agent of historical importance.

Cushing's Reflex
The systemic vasoconstriction that occurs in response to an increased intracranial pressure (ICP). The resulting hypertension helps maintain cerebral perfusion pressure (CPP = MAP − ICP or CVP, whichever is higher). Baroreceptor mediated reflex bradycardia follows. The reflex is initiated by ischemia of medullary centers.

Cushing's syndrome
An endocrine disorder resulting from excessive amounts of glucocorticoids (primarily cortisol) in the blood. It also can be caused by medications or cortisol-producing tumors. Signs and symptoms are numerous and affect virtually every system in the body.

Cyanocobalamin
See pernicious anemia, vitamins, and cobalamins.

Cyanosis
The bluish coloration of the skin and/or mucous membranes; caused by increased levels of deoxygenated hemoglobin in the blood (more than 5g/dL). Common in certain congenital heart diseases, some abnormal hemoglobins, and nitrate poisoning.

Cyclins
Proteins that stimulate different phases of the cell cycle by activating enzymes called cyclin-dependent kinases.

Cyclooxygenase (COX)
An enzyme that promotes the formation of prostanoids (prostaglandins, thromboxanes and prostacyclin); it catalyzes the conversion of arachidonic acid to prostaglandin H_2, the precursor of all prostanoids. Two isoforms exist – COX-1 and COX-2. Non Steroidal Anti-inflammatory Drugs (NSAIDs) like aspirin, ibuprofen, and ketorolac are classic COX inhibitors and are potent analgesics (decreases peripheral prostaglandin synthesis). Acetaminophen is believed to be a centrally acting COX inhibitor. *Also see non-steroidal anti-inflammatory drugs, prostaglandins, and thromboxane.*

Cytochromes
Iron-containing proteins involved in oxidative phosphorylation; located on the inner mitochondrial membrane and are involved in electron transport.

Cytokine
Type of protein secreted by T-lymphocytes; attacks virally-infected cells and cancer cells.

Cytokinesis
Cytoplasmic division that occurs following the completion of nuclear division (mitosis).

Cytolysis
Also called "immune lysis." A process of disruption of bacteria or blood cells when combined with their specific antibodies, in the presence of complement.

Cytoplasm
The semi fluid material, excluding the nucleus, found within the plasma membrane.

Cytoskeleton
The structural protein framework of the cytoplasm; it comprises microtubules, intermediate filaments, and actin filaments.

D

D-cells   *See Delta cells.*

Dark Adaptation   The gradual increase in photoreceptor sensitivity upon entry into a dark environment. It is due to increased amounts of visual pigment in the photoreceptors.

Dark Current   The steady inward diffusion of Na^+ into the rods and cones when the photoreceptors are in a dark environment. Stimulation by light blocks the dark currents causing hyperpolarization of the photoreceptors.

Dead Space volume (V_D)   The volume of inspired air that does not participate in gas exchange. Anatomic dead space is the volume of the conducting airways (between the mouth, nose, and the terminal bronchioles). Physiologic dead space is the sum of the anatomic dead space and alveolar dead space (wasted ventilation). The anatomic dead space is approximately a person's weight in pounds. *Also see conducting and respiratory zones and tidal volume.*

Deafness (Hearing loss)   Impaired hearing. *Nerve or sensorineural deafness* is caused by dysfunction of the cochlea or auditory nerve. *Conduction deafness is* caused by impaired sound transmission to the cochlea. Many advanced treatments such as cochlear implants now exist for hearing impairment. *Also see Weber and Rinne's tests.*

Decerebrate Rigidity   A condition (usually in animals) associated with exaggerated extensor reflexes. Causes include (a) removal of inhibitory influences originating in the cerebral cortex, the caudate nucleus, and the cerebellum. (b) Maintained activity of facilitating pathways e.g. reticulospinal and vestibulospinal tracts.

Decompression Sickness   Occurs when divers emerge to the surface too rapidly. Decreased barometric pressure upon ascent to sea level causes formation of nitrogen (N_2) bubbles from the dissolved nitrogen. Blockage of blood vessels by the bubbles results in muscle and joint pains (the bends) or CNS disturbances. Paralysis and death can occur in severe cases. Other names for this condition are: the bends, caisson disease, and diver's disease. Treatment is by immediate recompression in a hyperbaric chamber followed by gradual decompression. The same phenomenon has been described in any situation of sudden depressurization.

Decubitus (Ulcer)

Pressure area, bed sore, skin opening, or skin breakdown. A discolored or open area of skin damage caused by prolonged pressure. Areas overlying bony prominences are most at risk for ulcer formation. Conditions associated with poor nutrition, poor circulation and poor sensation can predispose to its formation. It is a preventable condition and is considered by most as an indication of poor care.

Deep Vein Thrombosis (DVT)

A blood clot in a vein; located deep from the skin and most commonly seen in the calf, thigh and pelvis. DVT can occur after major surgical procedures and may lead to life-threatening pulmonary embolism (PE). *Also see anticoagulation.*

Defecation

Expulsion of fecal waste from the rectum through the anus; the process occurs involuntarily, via a reflex involving sacral parasympathetic nerves. It is also regulated voluntarily via conscious control of the external anal sphincters.

Defibrillation

The delivery of strong electric current to the chest to terminate cardiac fibrillation (caused by continuous recycling of electrical waves through the myocardium). This is an important step in certain types of cardiac arrest as early defibrillation is associated with a higher chance of survival. The device used for this is called a defibrillator.

Deglutition

The process by which food is propelled from the mouth into the stomach. It begins as a voluntary process in the mouth and continues as an involuntary (pharyngeal and esophageal phases) process once the bolus enters the pharynx.

Delayed Hypersensitivity

A local inflammatory skin response that occurs 12-24 hours after exposure to an antigen. It is mediated by sensitized T lymphocytes. Chronic transplant rejection is also mediated by this mechanism. *Also see hypersensitivity.*

Delta Cells

Somatostatin-secreting cells present in the islets of Langerhans. They are also called D-cells.

Delta Waves

EEG waves below 3.5 cycles per second; they occur in very deep sleep, in infancy, and in severe organic brain disease. *Also see electroencephalogram.*

Dendrites

Highly-branched neuronal fibers that carry electrical signals towards the cell body.

Dendritic Cells

Specialized cells found in lymph nodes and the spleen; act as antigen-presenting cells (APCs) for T lymphocytes activation. Function as regulators of the immune system.

Denervation Hypersensitivity

Enhanced neurotransmitter sensitivity of innervated organs following a period of interruption of their innervation. Occurs in skeletal and smooth muscles and other end organs and is believed to be the result of proliferation of new receptors (upregulation).

Dense Bodies

A component of the cytoskeleton of smooth muscle cells; they are the functional equivalents of the Z-lines present in skeletal muscles.

Dentin

Thick layer of bone-like substance constituting the hard tissues of the teeth and surrounding the pulp cavity; it is prone to rapid decay from poor oral hygiene resulting in caries.

Deoxyhemoglobin

The form of hemoglobin that is devoid of oxygen. Also called reduced hemoglobin. *Also see hemoglobin.*

Deoxyribose

A five-carbon sugar present in DNA.

Depolarization

Applicable to excitable tissues; it involves a reduction or reversal of the normal polarization of the cell membrane. It is the initial phase of the action potential. *Also see action potential and repolarization.*

Depression

A form of mental illness associated with despair, misery, insomnia, loss of appetite, and decreased libido; probably caused by a decreased production of norepinephrine, serotonin or both, in the brain. *Also see affective disorders.*

Depressor Area

A region in the medulla that, upon stimulation, produces a decrease in blood pressure.

Descending Pathways

Consists of the pyramidal and extrapyramidal tracts. Pyramidal tracts descend directly from the cerebral cortex to the spinal cord without synaptic interruption. The extrapyramidal tracts originate in the medulla and brain stem and have numerous synaptic interconnections. *Also see corticospinal and extrapyramidal tracts.*

Desensitization

Phenomenon in which prolonged exposure to a substance e.g. a polypeptide hormone, reduces the responsiveness of the target cells upon subsequent exposure to the same concentration of the hormone. Also called down regulation or adaptation. May explain the decreased responsiveness to certain drugs after prolonged use, especially adrenergic drugs.

Desmin

Protein polymers present in intermediate filaments of smooth muscles. *Also see intermediate filaments.*

Detoxification

A metabolic process that occurs largely in the liver that involves chemical transformation to remove toxic components of molecules. It involves such processes as oxidation, hydrolysis, reduction, or conjugation. The term may also be used to refer to the treatment of drug addiction.

Detrusor muscle

The muscular wall of the urinary bladder.

Deuteranopia

A form of color blindness in which there is loss of the medium wavelength cone mechanism.

Developmental Disability

A broad term used to describe any mental and/or physical disability that has an onset before adulthood and usually lasting throughout life and associated with limitations in major life activities. It includes individuals with mental retardation, cerebral palsy, autism, epilepsy (and other seizure disorders), sensory impairments, congenital anomalies, disabilities caused by trauma or conditions caused by certain neurologic diseases.

Dexamethasone

A synthetic glucocorticoid that is about 30 times more potent than cortisol. A commonly used steroid in clinical practice.

Diabetes Insipidus

A condition in which there is a deficiency of antidiuretic hormone (ADH) secretion by the posterior pituitary (central type) or resistance of the kidneys to ADH (nephrogenic type). It is associated with inability to produce concentrated urine. *Also see antidiuretic hormone.*

Diabetes Mellitus

A group of disorders characterized by a high blood glucose level (hyperglycemia) and the appearance of glucose in the urine. It is due to an absolute or relative lack of insulin. There are two types: Insulin-dependent (Type I) and non-insulin dependent (Type II). It affects virtually every organ system in the body and is a significant cause of morbidity and mortality.

Dialysis

A process for clearing the blood of unwanted toxic materials. It usually involves selective diffusion through a porous membrane and ultrafiltration. Commonly used in the treatment of end stage renal disease (ESRD) and certain drug overdoses.

Diapedesis

A phenomenon in which leukocytes squeeze through the endothelial walls of capillaries.

Diarrhea

An increased frequency of watery stool from multiple etiologies; associated with severe loss of extracellular-type fluid; in extreme conditions may result in circulatory collapse from decreased intravascular volume. Excessive loss of bicarbonate ions in diarrheal stool can cause metabolic acidosis. It is a common cause of death in developing countries, especially in infants and small children.

Diaschisis

A theoretical state following brain injury in which healthy areas that are neuronally connected to the damaged area show a temporary loss of function.

Diastasis

The phase of the cardiac cycle characterized by slow ventricular filling. It follows the phase of rapid ventricular filling.

Diastole

The phase of relaxation during the cardiac cycle in which the ventricles refill with blood. It is the period between the second and first heart sounds. Most of the coronary blood flow occurs during this period. An excessive heart rate (tachycardia) decreases diastolic filling time and blood flow while increasing myocardial oxygen demand. Myocardial ischemia or infarction can occur in susceptible individuals. *Also see systole.*

Diastolic Blood Pressure

The lowest arterial blood pressure during the diastolic phase of the cardiac cycle. It is indicated by the last sound of Korotkoff when blood pressure is measured by auscultation. *Also see auscultatory blood pressure.*

Dichromat

Based on the trichromacy theory of color blindness; dichromats are individuals who lack one of the cone mechanisms.

Diencephalon

A component of the forebrain that encircles the third ventricle. It contains the hypothalamus, thalamus, and the pineal gland.

Diffuse Axonal Injury (DAI)

A shearing injury of large nerve fibers (axons covered with myelin) in many areas of the brain. It appears to be one of the two primary lesions of traumatic brain injury (TBI), the other being stretching or shearing of blood vessels from the same forces, producing hemorrhage. It is the leading cause of neurologic devastation following TBI.

Diffuse Brain Injury

Injury to cells in many areas of the brain rather than in a specific location (focal). A common finding in traumatic brain injury. Both diffuse and focal lesions commonly occur together.

Diffusion

The random movement of molecules or ions from regions of higher to regions of lower concentration.

Digestion

The process by which food is broken down into small molecules that can be readily absorbed.

Digitalis

A cardiotonic drug employed in the treatment of congestive heart failure and some arrhythmias; it increases heart muscle contraction and decreases heart rate. It is also called digoxin.

Dihydrotestosterone (DHT)

A biologically active metabolite of testosterone formed predominantly in the prostate gland. It is formed by the action of 5α-reductase. DHT stimulates the development of male characteristics. Congenital absence of this enzyme results in a failure to develop these features.

1, 25-Dihydroxycholecalciferol

The most active metabolite of vitamin D; it is produced by hydroxylation of vitamin D3 in the liver and kidney; it enhances intestinal absorption of Ca^{2+}.

Diltiazem

A calcium channel blocking drug. *Also see calcium channel blockers.*

Diplegia

Paralysis of corresponding parts on both sides of the body, such as both arms.

Diploid

A term denoting a cell having a full set of genetic material, with two of each kind of chromosome (one set donated from each parent) and not including the sex chromosomes. Humans have 22 pairs of matching chromosomes (autosomes) and 1 pair of sex chromosomes. This gives a diploid number of 46.

Diplopia

Seeing two images of a single object. Also called double vision.

Disability

Inability or limitation in performing tasks, activities, and roles in a manner or within the range considered normal. It may refer to a physical, mental or sensory condition.

Disaccharide

A sugar that contains two monosaccharide units; sucrose is an example.

Discrimination (Auditory)

The ability to differentiate and recognize sounds. This involves distinguishing between words, noises, and sounds that might be similar. A person with poor auditory discrimination might answer the phone in his room although the actual ringing came from an alarm clock.

Discrimination, Sensory

A process requiring differentiation of two or more stimuli.

Discrimination, Tactile

The ability to identify and distinguish between objects and stimuli solely by touch. It involves the ability to ascertain shape, size, and texture. For example, persons with impaired tactile discrimination may be unable to distinguish between different coins in their pocket.

Discrimination, Visual

Involves the differentiation of items using sight. Persons with impaired visual discrimination may not be able to distinguish between red and green light while driving. They may also have difficulty distinguishing the letter "E" from "F."

Disinhibition

Inability to suppress (inhibit) impulsive behavior and emotions.

Distal

Far from the point of reference.

Diuretic

A drug that increases urine production (*diuresis*). Most act by inhibiting Na^+ reabsorption in different parts of the nephron with reduction in water reabsorption. Some, like mannitol, act by their osmotic effect. Diuretics are used in renal disease, as antihypertensives, in heart failure, and to lower intracranial and intraocular pressures.

DNA (Deoxyribonucleic Acid)

Nucleic acid found in cells, composed of nucleotide bases and deoxyribose sugar. It contains the genetic code. *Also see double helix.*

DOPA (Dihydroxyphenylalanine)

Amino acid formed in the liver from tyrosine and converted to dopamine in the brain. L-dopa (used in the treatment of Parkinson's disease) stimulates dopamine production.

Dopamine

A central nervous system neurotransmitter; it is also the precursor of the neurotransmitter noradrenaline (norepinephrine) and adrenaline (epinephrine). Loss of brain dopamine is implicated in Parkinson's disease. Dopamine is also a commonly used inotrope in clinical practice.

Dopaminergic Pathways

Neural pathways in the brain that release dopamine; there are four main pathways:

- The nigrostriatal pathway – transmits dopamine from the substantia nigra to the striatum. It is involved in motor control; degeneration is related to Parkinson's disease.
- The mesocortical pathway – transmits dopamine from the ventral tegmental area to the frontal cortex. Lesions in this pathway result in schizophrenia.
- The mesolimbic pathway - transmits dopamine from ventral tegmental area to the nucleus accumbens.
- The tuberoinfundibular pathway – Transmits dopamine from the hypothalamus to the pituitary gland. It regulates the secretion of some hormones e.g. prolactin.

Doppler Blood Flow Measurement

A method for ultrasonic measurement of rapid and pulsatile blood flow; it involves the application of a flow detector over the blood vessel. The change in frequency as the sound waves are reflected by the red cells is proportional to the flow rate. Other applications of the Doppler effect include cardiac output measurement and fetal heart rate monitoring.

Dorsal Root Ganglion

Bundle of cell bodies of sensory neurons located in the dorsal root of a spinal nerve.

Dorsiflexion

To bend or flex toward the extensor part of a limb as in the foot or hand.

Double Helix

The Watson and Crick model of DNA in which two polynucleotide chains are joined together by phosphate diesters; the bases project at right angles from the chain into the center axis. *Also see DNA.*

Down syndrome (Trisomy 21)

A common chromosomal abnormality resulting from a trisomy (extra copy) of chromosome 21. Formerly called *Mongolism*. Associated with characteristic facial features, variable mental delay, congenital heart defects, and airway anomalies.

Ductus Arteriosus

A blood vessel that connects the pulmonary artery directly to the aorta in fetal and early neonatal life. Functional closure occurs within 2-3 weeks of extra-uterine life. Failure to close results in a patent ductus arteriosus (PDA), which may require surgical closure. Prostaglandin E_1 plays a role in the maintenance of the ductal patency and is used in newborns with ductal dependent congenital heart lesions to maintain perfusion and oxygenation until a palliative or definitive procedure is performed.

Duodenocolic Reflex

An intrinsic reflex originating from the duodenum; it enhances colonic motility.

Dwarfism

A condition characterized by abnormally short stature. It is the result of growth hormone deficiency, certain syndromes, or genetic defects.

Dysarthria

Difficulty in forming or speaking words; it is due to weakness of the muscles required for speaking or disruption in the neuromotor stimulus patterns required for accuracy and velocity of speech.

Dysdiadochokinesia

An expression of ataxia, associated with extreme difficulty with supination and pronation of the arm.

Dyskinesia

Impaired bile secretion due to disturbances in the contractions of the muscles of the gallbladder, ducts, and the sphincter of Oddi.

Dyslexia

An inability to properly interpret written language despite normal vision. It is more common in males.

Dysmetria

An expression of ataxia in which there is a lack of cerebellar coordination and an error in judgment of movement to a desired position.

Dysphagia

Difficulty with swallowing from various mechanisms and causes. May involve difficulty in oral preparation for the swallow or moving material from the mouth to the stomach It is a prominent feature of esophageal disease.

Dyspnea

A subjective feeling of "shortness of breath." Difficulty with breathing.

Dystrophin

A protein associated with skeletal muscle membrane (sarcolemma). In patients with Duchenne muscular dystrophy, there is a defect in the dystrophin gene resulting in an abnormal dystrophin in the muscles. Progressive muscle wasting, cardiomyopathy, and respiratory insufficiency occur, usually resulting in death by the second or third decade.

E

ECG (Electrocardiogram)

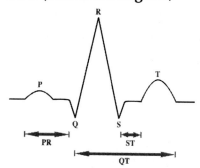

A surface recording of the heart's electrical activity. A useful test for various cardiac and certain electrolyte abnormalities. The P wave represents atrial depolarization, the QRS complex represents ventricular depolarization, and the T wave represents ventricular repolarization. Measurement of certain intervals and voltages on the ECG tracing provides useful information about abnormalities of cardiac function. *Also see QRS complex.*

Echocardiography

The diagnostic test utilizing ultrasound waves to acquire images of different aspects of the heart. Widely used for diagnosis of various heart conditions, especially valvular heart disease, wall motion abnormalities, myocardial function, and congenital heart diseases. Acquisition of measured and derived variables provides useful information about myocardial function.

Eclampsia

Convulsions (seizures) associated with pregnancy-induced hypertension. A very serious and life-threatening obstetric emergency. *Also see pre-eclampsia.*

Ectopic Focus

An abnormal pacemaker located in an area of the heart other than the SA node. A cause of arrhythmias.

Ectopic Pregnancy

Development of the embryo in locations other than the uterine cavity. Most common site is in the fallopian tubes; it may also occur in the peritoneal cavity. A ruptured ectopic pregnancy is a gynecologic emergency.

EDCF

See Endothelium-derived contracting factors.

Edema

Swelling resulting from the accumulation of tissue fluid in the intercellular spaces. Mechanisms of edema include increased capillary pressure, decreased oncotic pressure, increased capillary permeability, and lymphatic obstruction. Common in renal disease, congestive heart failure, and liver disease. *Also see colloid osmotic pressure, ascites, and Starling forces.*

EDHF

See Endothelium-derived hyperpolarizing factor.

Edinger-Westfall Nucleus

This is the visceral nucleus of the third cranial nerve (oculomotor), which passes into the ciliary ganglion. The parasympathetic preganglionic fibers arise from here.

It is located in the midbrain and is involved with the protection of the eye through the direct and consensual light reflexes.

EDRF

Denotes *Endothelium-derived relaxing factor*; it is released by intact vascular endothelial cells and causes vasodilatation. EDRF has been identified as nitric oxide (NO). Prostacyclin is also an EDRF. *Also see nitric oxide, EDCF, and EDHF.*

EEG (Electroencephalogram)

See electroencephalogram.

Effector Organs

Refers to muscles and glands that are activated by efferent (motor) neurons.

Efferent

Conveying or transporting outward or away from center; e.g. efferent nerve fibers or efferent arterioles. *Also see afferent.*

Efferent Arteriole

Renal blood vessel which transports blood away from the glomerulus.

Eicosanoids

Derivatives of fatty acids and arachidonic acid; abundant in cell membranes. Examples include prostaglandins and leukotrienes. *Also see cyclooxygenase, prostaglandins, and non-steroidal anti-inflammatory drugs (NSAIDS).*

Einthoven's Triangle

An imaginary equilateral triangle used for the determination of the electrical axis of the ECG; the heart is located in the center while the three sides of the triangle represent the three standard limb leads of the electrocardiogram (I, II, III). *Also see precordial leads.*

EKG (Electrocardiogram)

Common usage in the United States. *See ECG.*

Elastic Fiber

Yellow fiber found in the matrix of connective tissues; possesses contractile properties and provides flexibility.

Elastic Recoil

A property of some muscles that make them return to their original position from a contraction or relaxation phase. Examples include: intrapulmonary airways during expiration and the aorta during protodiastole. It is decreased by advancing age and emphysema and increased in restrictive pulmonary disease.

Electrical Axis (Heart)

The direction of current flow during ventricular depolarization; it is about 59° but may differ in obese or lean subjects. It is determined from the mean QRS vector (a summation of the positive and negative deflections of an ECG). Axis deviation is seen in ventricular hypertrophy and bundle branch blocks. *Also see mean electrical axis.*

Electrical Synapses

These are junctions between nerves i.e. (axo-dendritic, axo-somatic, axo-axonic junctions) where transfer of information/impulse occurs through the depolarization of the post synaptic membrane by electric charges; e.g. gap junctions of intercalated disc found in cardiac muscle and giant squid axons. Electrical synapses transmit at high frequency with no delay; anoxia and metabolic inhibitors have little or no effect.

Electrocardiogram

See ECG.

Electrocorticogram

Measurement of electrical signals or potentials (mV) obtained with the use of electrodes placed directly on the pial surface of the cortex. This is an invasive procedure and a variation of this technique (subdural grids and strips) is used in the evaluation of patients with intractable seizures.

Electroencephalogram (EEG)

A recording of the electrical activity of the brain from surface electrodes placed on the scalp. First described by German psychiatrist Hans Berger; it denotes a recording of electrical signals or potentials (mV) obtained from the brain during various activities and stages of sleep. Based on differences in amplitude and frequency, they are classified as alpha, beta, theta rhythms and delta waves. A useful tool for detecting brain changes associated with epilepsy, sleep disorders, and metabolic brain disorders.

Electrogenic Na$^+$ Pump

A membrane pump that utilizes Na$^+$- K$^+$ ATPase to produce the energy needed for transport of three Na$^+$ out of the cell in exchange for two K$^+$. It produces a net loss of positive ions and it is an example of an antiport transport mechanism. *Also see antiport.*

Electromyogram (EMG)

A recording of the electrical activity of skeletal muscle using surface electrodes. In conjunction with measurements of nerve conduction, it is useful in diagnosing nerve, muscle, and neuromuscular disorders.

Electrophoresis

A biochemical technique in which charged particles in

a colloid undergo movement under the influence of an electric field. A very useful technique in detecting abnormal proteins in conditions such as monoclonal gammopathy, multiple myeloma, and sickle hemoglobin. Gel electrophoresis is a very useful method for DNA and RNA separation and research with implications for wide application in medical research and forensic medicine.

Elephantiasis

A disease caused by the larvae of nematode parasitic worms. The larvae invade and block lymphatic vessels producing lymphedema and an elephant-like appearance. Common in Africa, Asia, the Pacific, the Americas, and South East Asia.

Embolus

Blood clot, or any other material, that is carried in the blood stream to other sites causing obstruction to flow. Air, fat, amniotic fluid and tumor emboli are other examples. Pulmonary embolus is a common example and significant cardiovascular compromise can occur in severe cases. *Also see thrombus.*

EMG

See Electromyogram.

Emmetropia

Denotes a condition of normal refractive vision; the image of an object is focused clearly on the retina.

Emphysema (pulmonary)

A lung disease associated with increased air spaces (over inflation). Forced vital capacity is decreased and airway resistance increased. In combination with chronic bronchitis, constitute the syndrome called Chronic obstructive pulmonary disease (COPD).

Emulsification

The process by which large fat globules are broken down into smaller units by the detergent action of bile salts.

End-Diastolic Volume (EDV)

The volume of blood in the ventricles at the end of diastole. Normal adult value is 130 mL. 65% of this is ejected with each stroke (ejection fraction). Clinically, this volume is estimated by measuring the filling pressures of the right and left heart by measuring central venous pressure and the pulmonary artery wedge pressure, respectively. *Also see end systolic volume.*

Endocrine Glands

Ductless glands; glands that secrete hormones directly into the blood stream rather than into a duct.

Endocytosis

A process which occurs by invagination of the cell membrane; the membrane fuses, allowing a small vesicle containing extracellular fluid to be pinched off, and enter the cell. This process allows cellular uptake of large molecules such as proteins.

Endoderm

The innermost of the primary tissue layer of the embryo. It is formed in the third week of gestation and gives rise to the linings of the gastrointestinal tract, the respiratory tract, the bladder, liver, gall bladder, pancreas, parathyroid, thymus glands and the urethra. The other two layers are ectoderm and mesoderm.

Endogenous

Produced within an organism.

Endolymph

Fluid contained within the membranous labyrinth of the inner ear. It is similar in composition to intracellular fluid.

Endometriosis

Presence of endometrial tissue outside the uterus such as in the pelvic cavity or other sites in the abdomen. A common cause of gynecological complaints such as pelvic pain.

Endometrium

The mucous membrane lining of the uterus; it is made up of two layers: basal layer and an inner functional layer. The endometrium participates in the formation of the placenta.

Endomysium

The sheath of connective tissue that surrounds each muscle fiber. Perimysium surrounds each fascicle or group of muscle fibers, while the epimysium encases the muscles.

Endopeptidases

Enzymes secreted from the small intestine that split smaller peptides into amino acids. Include chymotrypsin, trypsin, elastase, and amino peptidases. They act on interior (non-terminal) peptide bonds.

Endoperoxides

Chemical intermediates in the activity of a variety of bioactive agents e.g. prostaglandins and artemisinin.

Endoplasmic Reticulum (ER)

A complicated system of membranous channels and flattened vesicles; physically continuous with the outer nuclear membrane. There are two types of ER: smooth and rough ER. They are involved in protein, lipid, and steroid synthesis as well as calcium regulation. *Also see sarcoplasmic reticulum.*

Endorphins

Special endogenous opioid neurotransmitters found in the brain; act as natural analgesic agents and produce a feeling of tranquility. Other opioid peptides are enkephalins and dynorphins. *Also see enkephalins.*

Endothelial Cell Growth Factor

A protein growth factor that exists in many isoforms; involved in new blood and lymphatic vessel formation. Two target receptors have been identified as tyrosine kinases. Attempts to block their actions are a central focus of anti-angiogenesis research that may eventually translate to advances in cancer treatment. *Also see angiogenesis.*

Endothelin

A 21 amino acid polypeptide similar in sequence to the safarotoxins produced by a snake (*Atractaspis engaddensis*). Endothelin-1 is secreted by the endothelium of blood vessels and is the most potent vasoconstrictor known; it acts on two types of receptors: ET_A and ET_B. The other forms of endothelin (ET-2 and ET-3) are of unknown origin.

Endothelium

The innermost layer of the tunica interna of the walls of arteries and veins; composed of simple squamous epithelium.

Endothelium-derived contracting factors (EDCF)

Vasoconstrictor agents usually produced by damaged vascular endothelial cells. May play a role in the causation of hypertension and atherosclerosis. *Also see nitric oxide and EDHF.*

Endothelium-derived hyperpolarizing factor (EDHF)

A vasorelaxant produced by vascular endothelial cells; it produces hyperpolarization of vascular smooth muscle cells.

Endotoxin

A lipopolysaccharide present in the cell walls of gram-negative bacteria which stimulates monocytes and macrophages to release cytokines. The cytokines, mainly interleukin-1, interleukin-6 and tumor necrosis factor (TNF), induce fever, sleepiness and a fall in plasma levels of iron. They are extremely toxic and may be involved in the causation of septic shock.

End-Plate Potential (EPP)

See motor endplate potential.

End-Systolic Volume

The volume of blood left in the ventricles after ventricular systole. *Also see end diastolic volume.*

Enkephalins

Five amino acid polypeptide found in the brain. The two known enkephalins are met-enkephalin and leu-enkephalin. They possess analgesic properties and also function as brain neurotransmitters and neuromodulators. *Also see endorphins.*

Enteric Nervous System

A term referring to the neuronal network of the intestine.

Enteritis

Infections of the gastrointestinal tract; one of the causes of diarrhea and cholera which leads to loss of ions, fluid and nutrients. It can also be caused by pantothenic acid deficiency.

Enterochromaffin-Like (ECL) Cells

Histamine-secreting cells present in gastric glands. They are stimulated by gastrin and vagal activity.

Enterocytes

Epithelial cells located in the superficial layer of the small and large intestines; involved in the breaking down and transport of molecules into tissue.

Enteroglucagon

A glucagon-like polypeptide secreted by the ileum and the colon; it stimulates insulin secretion, raises blood glucose level and inhibits gastrointestinal motility. It is immunologically distinct from pancreatic glucagon. *Also see glucagon.*

Enterohepatic Circulation

The recirculation of bile between the liver and small intestine via the hepatic portal vein.

Enterokinase

Also known as enteropeptidase; it converts the inactive trypsinogen to active trypsin and is secreted by the duodenal mucosa. Its secretion is increased by cholecystokinin.

Enteropathy

Any disease of the intestinal tract.

Enzyme

A protein catalyst for specific chemical reactions.

Eosinophil

A type of white blood cell that contains cytoplasmic granules, which stain with eosin or other acidic dyes.

Ephaptic Transmission

Transmission across artificial synapses called ephapses.

Epidermal Growth Factor

A polypeptide growth factor which stimulates the *in vitro* proliferation of various cell types; it is involved in the induction of mitosis.

Epidermis

Layer of the skin, composed of stratified squamous epithelium; the outer layer is non-functional and is filled with keratin.

Epididymis	A tubular structure outside the testes which serves as a site for the storage and maturation of spermatozoa between ejaculations.
Epilepsy	A central nervous system (CNS) dysfunction characterized by: uncontrolled, paroxysmal, and excessive activity of either a part or all of the CNS. Usually results in generalized convulsions, autonomic, and sensory disturbances as well as impairment of consciousness. Various types have been described.
Epinephrine	*See Adrenaline.*
Episome	A genetic material (DNA) in bacteria that can replicate separately inside the main bacterial chromosome; e.g. plasmids.
Epithelium	Type of membranous tissue that covers internal and external surfaces of the body including blood vessels and cavities.
EPSP (Excitatory Postsynaptic Potential)	A transient and graded depolarization of a postsynaptic neuron as a result of an action potential in a presynaptic cell. EPSPs can undergo summation.
Equilibrium Potential	The theoretical membrane potential that would be produced if the membrane were permeable to only one ion. The equilibrium potential for an ion can be derived using the Nernst equation: the value for Na^+, with extracellular and intracellular concentrations of 145 mEq/L and 12 mEq/l, respectively is + 60mV. *Also see Nernst equation.*
Equatorial division	The second meiotic (nuclear) division in which the number of chromosomes remains unchanged.
Erection	This is a reproductive reflex action under the control of the parasympathetic nervous system. It occurs when blood fills the spongy tissues of the penis through the penile artery following sexual arousal. Failure of this mechanism is the cause of erectile dysfunction (ED) and is treated by agents that increase blood flow. *Also see nitric oxide.*
Eructation	*See belching.*
Erythroblast	The stage after the pluripotential stem cell in the erythrocytes formation process; the RBC contains a nucleus during this stage. *Also see erythrocyte.*

Erythroblastosis Fetalis

Severe hemolytic disease of the newborn; hemolysis of the Rh-positive RBCs of the newborn due to maternal anti-Rh antibodies. Mother is Rh-negative but develops anti-Rh antibodies from a prior exposure to Rh-positive cells in a previous pregnancy (sensitization). The anti-Rh antibodies can then attack a subsequent Rhesus positive fetus causing severe hemolytic disease. Anemia, heart failure, edema and jaundice are the hallmarks of severe cases (Hydrops Fetalis) and in utero fetal demise may occur. Prevention of maternal sensitization is by giving the mother Rh immune globulin [RhoGAM, IgG anti-D (anti-Rh)] to suppress the immune response to any Rh-positive red blood cells in her circulation.

Erythrocyte (red blood cell)

A red blood cell that is biconcave shaped and lacks a nucleus (in its mature form). Erythrocytes contain hemoglobin and transport oxygen to the tissues. *Also see erythroblast.*

Erythropoiesis

The process of red blood cell formation from the pluripotential stem cells to the mature red blood cells; occurs in the spleen and bone marrow in the fetus and newborns but only in the bone marrow beyond that. It is stimulated by hypoxia, hemorrhage, and anemia. Enhanced in the presence of the hormone erythropoietin. *Also see hematopoiesis.*

Erythropoietin

A polypeptide hormone secreted by the juxtaglomerular cells of the kidneys and stimulates the production of red blood cells by the bone marrow. Recombinant human erythropoietin (Epogen) is used in the treatment of anemia, especially those associated with chemotherapy.

Escherichia Coli

A bacteria species abundant in the human intestine. Pathologic forms are a common cause of food poisoning. Commonly called E. Coli.

Essential Amino Acids (EAAs)

Amino acids which the body requires but cannot make. There are eight amino acids in adults (nine in children). They are obtained from dietary sources. The EAAs are: Valine, Leucine, Isoleucine, Threonine, Methionine, Phenylalanine, Arginine, Lysine, and Histidine.

Esters (Phorbol)

Polycyclic esters that irreversibly activate protein kinase C; isolated from croton oil. An example is: 12-O-tetradecanoyl-phorbol-13-acetate (TPA).

Estradiol

The principal estrogen secreted by the ovaries.

Estrogen

The female hormone also called Estradiol; produced under the influence of follicle stimulating hormone (FSH) in the ovarian follicle and corpus luteum. It stimulates the thickening of the uterine wall, maturation of the oocyte, development of the female sex characteristics and increases luteinizing hormone (LH) secretion. Inhibition of FSH occurs through a negative feedback mechanism.

Estrus Cycle

A term applicable to non-primate female mammals whereby sexual receptivity occurs at a particular time of their "menstrual" cycles. Involves cyclic changes in the structure and function of the ovaries

Excitation-Contraction Coupling

The series of events that link the excitation of a muscle membrane to muscle contraction. E-C coupling involves the transduction of a membrane signal to an intracellular contractile machinery using intracellular free calcium ions $[Ca^{2+}]_i$ as a second messenger.

Excitatory Amino Acid

Amino acids that function as neurotransmitters in the central nervous system; examples include glutamate and aspartate; they evoke EPSPs in brain neuron. Glycine is excitatory in the brain but inhibitory in other sites in the nervous system while GABA is inhibitory. Anesthetic action is believed to be due to enhancement of inhibitory pathways in the brain, especially GABA, and inhibition of excitatory pathways.

Excretion

The process of disposal of metabolic wastes.

Exergonic

Denoting chemical reactions that liberate energy.

Exocrine Gland

A gland that releases its secretion through a duct; examples include sweat gland and salivary gland.

Exocytosis

The process of cellular secretion or excretion in which the substances contained within cellular vesicles are released from the cell by fusion of the vesicular membrane with the cell membrane. This exposes the vesicular membrane to the extracellular medium.

Exon

A nucleotide sequence in DNA that defines a protein's DNA sequence by coding information that is transcribed to messenger RNA.

Expiration

The process of expulsion of air from the lungs.

Extensor

A muscle which extends or straightens part of the body, usually an extremity, when it contracts.

External Anal Sphincter

Sphincter located at the level of the anus and consists of skeletal muscle fibers. It enables conscious control of defecation.

Exteroceptor

A sensory receptor that responds to external stimuli; e.g. receptors on the skin.

Extracellular Fluid (ECF)

The fluid outside cells. It has two components: plasma and interstitial fluid. ECF makes up one third of total body water, corresponding to about 20% of body weight. The "Third Space" is a non-functional interstitial fluid compartment which expands following major trauma, burn injury, major surgery and other acute inflammatory conditions. It is believed to be an important cause of volume depletion in these settings and generally requires replacement.

Extrafusal Fibers

The ordinary muscle fibers which make up the bulk of the belly of skeletal muscles. *Also see intrafusal fibers.*

Extraocular Muscles

A group of six tiny muscles (comprising four rectus and two oblique muscles) which surround the eye and work in unison to control eye movement.

Extrapyramidal Tracts

Neural pathways situated outside of the pyramidal tracts. They form a part of the motor system involved in the coordination of movement. Signals start in the cortex and are relayed to the basal ganglia; from here, information is relayed to the red nucleus via the caudate, putamen, globus pallidus II (GPII) and globus pallidus I (GPI), the subthalamic nuclei and substantia nigra. Finally, information is relayed to the spinal cord via the rubrospinal tract. The extrapyramidal tracts are influenced by activity in the brain involving many synapses, and they appear to be required for fine control of voluntary movements. *Also see descending pathways and corticospinal tracts.*

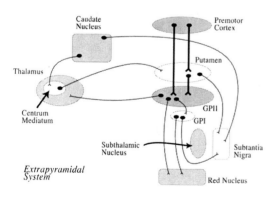

Extrasystole

Also known as a *premature beat*, it is a premature contraction of the heart that is not due to a normal sinus rhythm. Usually results from ectopic foci in the heart, ischemia, and toxins and during central venous and cardiac catheterization.

Extrinsic Nerves

Nerves involved in the control of events in an organ or tissue that are distinct from the intrinsic or internally-mediated control system. The vagus nerve is an example of an extrinsic nerve to the gastrointestinal tract.

F

Facilitated Diffusion	A form of carrier-mediated transport of molecules through the cell membrane. The process does not require energy (ATP) as molecules or ions are carried down a concentration gradient.
Facilitation	A phenomenon by which repeated stimulation of a presynaptic axon results in enhanced postsynaptic response with each stimulus; the degree of facilitation depends on the frequency of presynaptic impulses. Post-tetanic potentiation (PTP) of skeletal muscle contraction is due to massive release of acetylcholine quanta prior to a single twitch contraction. This form of facilitation is employed as a useful test of neuromuscular function.
FAD (Flavin Adenine Dinucleotide)	A cofactor in the following enzymes: D-amino acid oxidase, glucose oxidase, and xanthine oxidase. It is obtained from riboflavin and plays a role in mitochondrial electron transport.
Farsightedness	*See hyperopia.*
Fasciculation	The contraction of whole motor unit following an abnormal impulse in a motor nerve fiber. It occurs especially following destruction of the anterior motor neurons e.g. in poliomyelitis. Fasciculations are also seen with depolarizing muscle relaxants such as succinylcholine.
Fasting	Food deprivation; associated with this is a reduction in blood glucose level.
Fat Cells	These are modified fibroblasts of adipose tissues capable of storing almost pure triglycerides in quantities equal to 80% to 95% of their volumes; they can also synthesize small amounts of fatty acids and triglycerides from carbohydrates.
Fat-Soluble Vitamins	Includes Vitamin A (carotene), Vitamin D (cholecalciferol), Vitamin E (Tocopherols) and Vitamin K (phylloguinone). They are commonly referred to as the ADEK vitamins. *Also see vitamins.*
Feces	The solid excretory product released from the large intestine.

Feedback

A mechanism through which an action is regulated by sending impulses back to its initiator e.g. the negative and positive feedback mechanisms in the control of homeostatic functions. *Also see negative feedback.*

Ferritin

The iron-apoferritin complex that is involved in iron (Fe) transport from the intestine to the plasma. Transferrin, a β-globulin, is also involved. *Also see transferrin.*

Fertility

Being productive/reproductive or non-sterile.

Fertilization

The process leading to the formation of a zygote through the combination of the spermatozoa and ovum.

Fetal Distress Syndrome

An abnormal state of a fetus associated with altered heart rate or rhythm, resulting from impaired oxygen delivery to the fetus. This term is now rarely used because of the unfavorable medico-legal connotation and terms such as "non-reassuring fetal heart rate" are now commonly used.

Fetal Hemoglobin (HbF)

The type of hemoglobin found in the fetus. It consists of 2α and 2γ chains unlike the adult that consists of 2α and 2β chains. Has more affinity for oxygen because of the loose binding to 2,3-DPG (diphosphoplycerate). The oxyhemoglobin dissociation curve (OHDC) is shifted to the left. It accounts for 80% of hemoglobin at birth and usually disappears completely by six months of life. *Also see sickle cell anemia.*

Fetal Alcohol Syndrome (FAS)

A condition associated with excessive alcohol consumption during pregnancy. FAS infants exhibit growth retardation, facial or neural abnormalities, cardiac defects and other developmental defects. Occurs in 1-2 infants/1000 live births.

Fever (Pyrexia)

An elevation of body temperature above the normal daily variation. Normal body temperature at rest taken under the tongue is $36.7 \pm 0.6\ ^0C$. There is elevation of the hypothalamic set-point, which results in a vasomotor response and shivering in order to achieve a new set point. Antipyretic agents such as acetaminophen (paracetamol) and aspirin reduce fever by resetting the set point thus producing sweating and peripheral vasodilatation. Fever is a very common symptom and sign that has numerous etiologies (infectious and non-infectious). *Also see hyperpyrexia.*

Fiber	*See Muscle Fiber and Nerve.*
Fibrillation	A cardiovascular dysfunction associated with abnormal heart rhythm and a low cardiac output due to activity of ectopic foci or myocardial infarction. Ventricular Fibrillation (VF) is a life-threatening emergency that requires immediate defibrillation. *Also see defibrillation.*
Fibrin	Produced from fibrinogen by the action of thrombin; it forms a mesh (fibrin clot) which covers an injury site and prevents excessive bleeding.
Fibrinogen	Factor II in the coagulation cascade; it is converted to fibrin monomer/threads by the action of thrombin.
Fibrinolysin (Plasmin)	The proteolytic enzyme that digests fibrin fibers and other clotting factors. Formed from plasminogen, by the action of thrombin and tissue plasminogen activator (t-PA). Recombinant t-PA is used clinically in the treatment of acute myocardial infarction to lyse clots in the coronary arteries. t-PA is also used to lyse clots in different parts of the body especially in the field of interventional radiology. *Also see tissue plasminogen activators and thrombin.*
Fibrinolysis (Fibrinolytic System)	The process by which fibrin clots are degraded by plasmin in order to restore normal blood flow. Fibrin degradation products (now called D-Dimers) act alongside the clotting system to prevent excessive intravascular coagulation. Abnormal activation of the coagulation and fibrinolytic systems in certain disease states results in a very serious condition called disseminated intravascular coagulopathy (DIC). Antifibrinolytic agents such as aminocaproic acid, tranexamic acid and aprotinin inhibit the proteolytic effect of plasmin on fibrin thus promoting coagulation and decreasing bleeding. These drugs are used during cardiopulmonary bypass, liver transplantation and certain orthopedic procedures to decrease bleeding and the need for donor blood transfusion. Aprotinin has recently been withdrawn due to reports of serious complications. *Also see streptokinase.*
Fibroblast Growth Factor	A type of growth factor that stimulates angiogenesis; it also stimulates bone formation and calcium metabolism.

Fick Principle

A method for cardiac output (CO) measurement based on an application of the law of mass conservation: the amount of blood flowing through the lungs per minute (which is equivalent to the cardiac output) is calculated as follows:

$$CO \text{ (L/min)} = \frac{O_2 \text{ consumption mL/ min by the lungs}}{\text{Arteriovenous } O_2 \text{ difference (mL/liter)}}$$

Also see appendix I.

Fight or Flight Response

A reaction also called *mass action*; associated with increased sympathetic discharge (release of norepinephrine and epinephrine from the adrenal medulla) under stressful conditions.

Flaccid Paralysis

Loss of muscle tone resulting from failure of muscles to contract. Causes include: lower motor neuron damage and failure of neuromuscular transmission.

Flagellum

Slender structure that propels a cell (e.g. spermatozoa) through a fluid medium.

Flare-and-Wheal Reaction

See triple response.

Flavoprotein

A conjugated protein that participates in electron transport within the mitochondria.

Flexion Reflex

A reflex action leading to flexion e.g. ankle jerk and biceps jerk.

Flexor

A muscle that, upon contraction, flexes a joint.

Follicle Stimulating Hormone (FSH)

A gonadotropin released from the anterior pituitary under the influence of gonadotropin releasing hormone. It stimulates growth of ovarian follicles, ovulation in females, and sperm production in males. *Also see gonadotropic hormones.*

Fontanel

Membranous spaces between cranial bones; they close during the course of normal development. The anterior and posterior are the major fontanels. A bulging fontanel may suggest a raised intracranial pressure (ICP) from various causes. A sunken fontanel is usually indicative of a low ICP commonly caused by dehydration.

Food Intake (Regulation)

Ingestion of food; regulation is under the influence of the hypothalamus: the hypothalamus has a feeding center (which regulates food intake) and the satiety

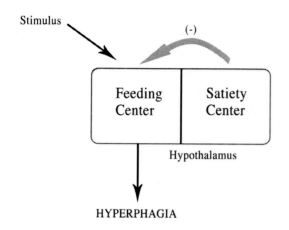

Stimulus

(-)

Feeding Center | Satiety Center

Hypothalamus

HYPERPHAGIA

center (which signals satisfaction by sending inhibitory signals to the feeding center). The feeding and satiety centers contain neurons with receptors sensitive to a wide variety of neurotransmitters: those that decrease feeding, e.g. serotonin, norepinephrine, leptin and those that stimulate feeding e.g. neuropeptide Y (NPY), endorphins, some amino acids [glutamate, gamma amino butyric acid (GABA)]. Food intake is regulated on short- and long-term basis. Short-term regulation prevents overeating by (a) Gastric Filling – inhibitory signals are sent to the feeding center; GIT filling also induces the release of hormones e.g. cholecystokinin, glucagons and insulin which inhibit the feeding center. (b) Oral Factors - by some yet undefined mechanisms, oral factors e.g. tasting, chewing, salivation and swallowing temporarily inhibit the feeding center. Long-term regulation involves the *glucostatic theory*: i.e. regulation of feeding by blood glucose level. Similar theories also exist for blood amino acid levels (aminostatic) and blood lipid levels (lipostatic). Decreased blood levels of these substances increase feeding, restoring normal levels. Increased blood glucose levels increase neuronal activity of the satiety center in the hypothalamus and thus decreases activity of neurons in the hunger center.

Foramen Magnum

Large opening in the occipital bone through which the spinal cord passes from the cranial cavity to the vertebral column.

Foramen Ovale

A small opening in the atrial septum that directs blood from the right atrium to the left atrium, bypassing the lungs, during fetal life. It closes at birth in most people but may persist in about 25% of the population (patent foramen ovale).

Forced Expiratory Volume (FEV$_1$)

A respiratory function test that measures the percentage of the forced vital capacity that is expired in the first second. A decreased ratio of FEV1/FVC suggests obstructive lung disease e.g. asthma. An increased ratio, usually due to a decreased FRC, is indicative of restrictive lung disease. *Also see forced vital capacity.*

Forced vital capacity (FVC)

The amount of air that can be forcibly expelled after a maximal inspiration. Measured by spirometry. *Also see forced expiratory volume (FEV$_1$) and spirometry.*

Fovea Centralis

A depressed area in the yellowish spot on the retina (macula lutea); it contains only cones and has the highest acuity for both images and color vision. *Also see macula lutea.*

Frank-Starling law (of the heart)

This describes an intrinsic ability of the heart to adapt to changing volume loads (venous return); the greater the end-diastolic volume (greater stretch of the myocardium), the stronger the contraction produced. This principle has been used in the treatment of certain critically ill patients by measuring their cardiac output (CO) at different preloads (plotting their Starling's curve), until CO and oxygen delivery are optimized. *Also see Appendix I.*

Functional Hyperemia

Also called active hyperemia; denotes the increase in blood flow to various organs due to an increase in metabolic activity in such organs or tissues. The increase in blood flow caused by increased metabolic activity is very high in skeletal muscles during exercise but moderate in the cerebral circulation. *Also see reactive hyperemia.*

Functional Residual Capacity (FRC)

A combination of the expiratory reserve volume and residual volume. FRC is about 2.2L in men and 1.8 L in females. It is the volume of air left in the lungs after normal expiration. It acts as an oxygen reservoir and factors that reduce it such as supine position, obesity, and pregnancy predispose to hypoxemia. Certain methods of artificial ventilation increase or maintain FRC thus improving oxygenation.

G

G-Cells	Also called APUD (amine precursor uptake and decarboxylation) cells. They are located in the pyloric antral region of the stomach and they secrete gastrin.
G-Proteins	Guanine nucleotide binding proteins; these are nucleotide-regulatory proteins spanning the cell membrane that couple receptors with second messengers. G-proteins exist in two states: *activated* (with a higher affinity for GTP) and *inactivated* (with a higher affinity for GDP). They consist of α, β and γ subunits and are activated by G-protein-coupled receptors. G-proteins are involved in cellular signal transduction processes.
Galactose	A dietary carbohydrate; also a hexose polymer.
Galactorrhea	A condition of persistent lactation due to continuous prolactin release from prolactin-producing tumors. It is a cause of secondary infertility due to FSH and LH inhibition.
Gall Bladder	An organ associated with the liver; it stores and concentrates bile from the liver and releases it in response to the presence of fatty substances in the duodenum. The gall bladder empties in response to parasympathetic stimulation and the hormone cholecystokinin.
Gallstones	Stones or calculi formed in the gallbladder or bile duct due to the precipitation of certain substances e.g. calcium bilirubinate stones, cholesterol stones, etc. Gall stones (cholelithiasis) is a common indication for surgical removal of the gall bladder (cholecystectomy).
Gamete	A collective term for haploid germ cells: two gametes (sperm and ovum) combine during fertilization to form a zygote.
Gamma-Aminobutyric Acid (GABA)	An amino acid believed to function as an inhibitory neurotransmitter in the central nervous system. Two types of GABA receptors have been identified (A and B). Enhanced GABA transmission is believed to be the mechanism of action of certain sedative and anesthetic agents.
Gamma Globulin	A globulin fraction with a molecular mass of about 156,000 Dalton; functions as an antibody (immunoglobulin) that helps the body fight infections. *Also see immunoglobulins.*

Gamma Motor Neuron

A type of somatic motor neuron that innervates intrafusal fibers within the muscle spindles. *Also see intrafusal fibers.*

Ganglion Cells

Found in the retina; the bipolar cell synapses on the ganglion while the amacrine cells connect ganglion cells to one another at the inner plexiform layer.

Gap Junctions

Junctions that exist between cell membranes through which ions or charges can flow from one cell to another. They are present in visceral smooth muscle and cardiac muscle and are also regarded as low resistance bridges that serve as electrical synapses.

Gas Exchange

The exchange of gases (O_2 and CO_2) by the process of diffusion down their concentration gradients; e.g. between pulmonary capillaries and alveoli and between systemic capillaries and the surrounding tissue cells.

Gastric Acid

Hydrochloric acid, produced by parietal cells; it maintains the acidic pH of the stomach and aids the conversion of pepsinogen to active pepsin.

Gastric Emptying

Emptying of stomach contents into the duodenum; it is enhanced by the amount of food in the stomach, the intensity of antral peristaltic contractions, and gastrin. It is inhibited by duodenal factors e.g. fats, acidity, hypo- or hyper-tonicity etc. Gastric emptying is delayed in stressful situations such as trauma and burns, in diabetes mellitus and autonomic dysfunction. Metoclopramide increases gastric emptying (gastrokinetic effect) by a selective cholinergic effect.

Gastric Inhibitory Peptide (GIP)

Released from the upper small intestine in response to the presence of fat and carbohydrates in chyme. It stimulates the secretion of insulin by the pancreas and also inhibits gastric motility.

Gastric Intrinsic Factor

See Intrinsic factor.

Gastric Juice

Secretion containing water, hydrochloric acid, mucus and pepsinogen; produced by gastric glands.

Gastrin

A hormone secreted by the G-cells in the pyloric glands and the Brunner's glands in the duodenum. It exists in two forms G17 and G34. It enhances gastric secretion and motility. *Also see pentagastrin.*

Gastritis	Inflammation of the gastric mucosa by the presence of irritant foods, acids, or pathogens. Helicobacter pylori is a common cause of gastritis and ulcers. Treatment is with antacids, proton-pump inhibitors (omeprazole), antibiotics and removal of the offending agent. *Also see peptic ulcer and omeprazole.*
Gastro esophageal Sphincter	*See lower esophageal sphincter.*
Gastrocolic Reflex	A reflex which results from the distension of the stomach and facilitates mass movement in the colon. This explains defecation after feeds in small children.
Gastroileal Reflex	Gastric emptying causes relaxation of the ileocecal valve. It originates in the stomach and is mediated via the enteric nervous system. It produces increased ileal motility. *Also see ileogastric reflex.*
Gates	Chemically-regulated or voltage-regulated structures present in cell membranes for regulating ion movement through membrane channels. They are classified as ligand-gated or voltage gated based on their gating mechanism. They are also classified based on their ion selectivity. Also used to describe the *Gate control theory* of pain modulation by stimulation of large diameter pain fibers.
Gene Therapy	Application of genetic engineering or biotechnology for treatment of genetic and other diseases. It involves the transfer of genetically altered DNA into cells with transcription of the recombinant gene, which corrects the genetic defect. Cystic fibrosis, hemophilia and certain cancers are potential applications for this therapy. *Also see knockout mice and p53.*
Generator Potential	The graded local depolarization produced in response to an environmental stimulus in a sensory receptor; it results in the production of action potentials by the sensory neuron.
Genetic Recombination	The process of formation of new combinations of genes, involving crossing-over between homologous chromosomes.
Genetic Transcription	The organic process by which the genetic code (DNA sequence) of bases is transferred from DNA to mRNA.

Genetic Translation

The process by which the amino acid sequence in messenger RNA is read by ribosomes to produce proteins.

Genome

The specific set of genes possessed by an individual, responsible for determining inherited characteristics; it also denotes the total set of genes that make up the characteristics of a species.

Gerontology

The study of the aging process.

Gibbs-Donnan Equilibrium

An equilibrium that exists as a result of movement of cations across the cell membrane.

Gigantism (Giantism)

A condition characterized by excessive growth in height resulting from excessive secretion of growth hormone in adolescence. *Also see acromegaly and growth hormone.*

Glaucoma

An eye disorder characterized by a raised intraocular pressure (IOP). Usually caused by obstruction of the canal of Schlemm (for the reabsorption of the aqueous humor). Two types: open angle and angle closure glaucoma. Common with advancing age but also seen in children. May progress to blindness if IOP is not controlled.

Glial Cells (Neuroglia)

Non-neuronal cells found mainly in the central nervous system; there are two types: microglia and macroglia. Microglia are specialized macrophages and macroglia consist of two main types: oligodendrocytes, which produce the myelin sheath of axons, and astrocytes (with characteristic star-like appearance), which provide mechanical and metabolic support to neurons. *Also see astrocytes and Schwann cells.*

Globulin

See gamma globulin.

Glomerular Filtration Rate (GFR)

The volume of glomerular ultrafiltrate produced by the kidneys per minute; GFR is measured by the renal plasma clearance of inulin; its normal value is about 125 mL/min. *See inulin and renal clearance.*

Glomerular Ultrafiltrate

The fluid formed by the hydrostatic pressure of blood entering the Bowman's capsule.

Glomeruli

The network of capillaries responsible for producing the blood filtrate that enters the renal tubules.

Glomerulonephritis

A group of diseases associated with inflammation of the renal glomeruli; characterized by fluid retention, edema, hypertension and proteinuria and a deterioration of renal function. Autoimmune factors account for a majority of cases but infections may also be a causative factor.

Glottis
The structure responsible for vocalization in the larynx. It consists of the vocal cords and the aperture between them (rima glottidis). It is an important landmark for endotracheal intubation and is the narrowest part of the airway in adults. The cricoid cartilage is the narrowest part in children.

Glucagon
A 29-amino acid polypeptide hormone secreted by the alpha cells of the pancreatic islets of Langerhans; it stimulates glycogenolysis, lipolysis and the conversion of fatty acids to ketone bodies. *Also see enteroglucagon.*

Glucocorticoids
Any of a group of steroid hormones secreted by the adrenal cortex (corticosteroids) that specifically binds with cortisol receptors and influences the metabolism of carbohydrates, protein and fat resulting in an increase in blood glucose level. Glucocorticoids also have anti-inflammatory and immunosuppressant effects.

Glucokinase
A liver enzyme that phosphorylates glucose to glucose-6-phosphate; its activity is enhanced by insulin and attenuated by starvation and diabetes mellitus.

Gluconeogenesis
The conversion of non-carbohydrate molecules (e.g. amino acids and lactic acid), through pyruvic acid, to glucose.

Glucose
A hexose sugar and a principal product of carbohydrate metabolism. It is broken down during glycolysis and in the citric acid cycle (Kreb's cycle) for ATP production.

Glucoside
A glycoside in which glucose makes up the sugar constituent.

Glucosuria
See glycosuria.

GLUT (Proteins)
Transport carriers for the facilitated diffusion of glucose into cells. GLUT-1 transporter is expressed constitutively, increased by fasting and decreased by excess glucose; GLUT-4 is expressed in cardiac muscle, skeletal muscle, and adipose tissue.

Glutamate (Glutamic Acid)
The major excitatory neurotransmitter in the CNS; it is the ionized form of the amino acid, glutamic acid. It is also a major pain mediator.

Glycine

An amino acid which also functions as an inhibitory neurotransmitter in the central nervous system; it is released by certain spinal interneurons. Certain irrigation solutions used for urologic surgery contain glycine. Excessive absorption results in toxicity which can present as transient visual loss.

Glycogen

The storage form of glucose in humans; it is a polysaccharide of glucose - also called *animal starch* - produced primarily in the liver and skeletal muscles.

Glycogenesis

The formation of glycogen from glucose.

Glycogenolysis

The conversion of glycogen to glucose-6-phosphate; usually occurs in the liver in response to a low blood glucose.

Glycolysis

A metabolic pathway in the breakdown of glucose: conversion of glucose to two molecules of pyruvic acid. Glycolysis is associated with release of energy as hydrogen atoms are removed resulting in the formation of two ATP molecules.

Glycoproteins

Membrane proteins with covalently-bound carbohydrate side chains. Also called mucoproteins.

Glycosuria (Glucosuria)

The presence of glucose in the urine. Occurs when the transport maximum for glucose is exceeded. The most common cause is hyperglycemia from diabetes mellitus. May also occur during pregnancy due to a decreased renal threshold for glucose. Rarely, it is due to an intrinsic renal problem – renal glycosuria.

Goblet Cells

Mucus-secreting cells found in the gastrointestinal and respiratory tracts.

Goiter

An enlargement of the thyroid gland (hyperplasia) producing a neck mass. Causes include Grave's disease, Hashimoto's disease, Hyperthyroidism and iodine deficiency. *Also see Grave's disease and hyperthyroidism.*

Goldblatt Hypertension

Experimentally induced hypertension produced by clamping one renal artery. It is likely due to increased renin production as the kidney attempts to restore perfusion to normal levels. It is similar to clinical renal hypertension. It resolves by unclamping, use of ACE inhibitors, and nephrectomy (removal of the kidneys).

Golgi Apparatus

A complex network of membranous sacs located near the nucleus, within the cytoplasm of cells; it plays a role in the formation of glycoproteins, mucopolysaccharides and lysosomes.

Golgi Tendon Organ

Sensory receptor located in muscle tendons; detects changes in muscle tension. Also called neurotendinous receptor.

Gonadotropic Hormones

Hormones secreted by the anterior pituitary and the placenta that are responsible for stimulation of the ovaries and testes. They are: Follicle-stimulating hormone (FSH), Lutenizing hormone (LH), and human chorionic gonadotropin (hCG)- produced by the placenta during pregnancy. Detection of hCG is the basis of the urine or blood pregnancy test. A thorough understanding of the actions and functions of these hormones is the foundation for reproductive endocrinology, especially *in vitro* fertilization and other assisted reproductive technologies.

Gonads

A collective name for gamete-producing organs (testes and ovaries).

Graafian follicle

A mature ovarian follicle, consisting of one germ cell surrounded by a cluster of endocrine cells. Among other functions, it ensures the maturity of the oocyte, maintains hormonal support for the fetus and prepares the vagina and fallopian tubes for fertilization.

Grand Mal Seizures

Occurs in epilepsy and is characterized by extreme neuronal discharges in the brain, causing generalized tonic-clonic convulsions. *Also see epilepsy and petit mal seizures.*

Granular Leukocytes

Types of white blood cells (neutrophils, eosinophils, and basophils) characterized by the presence of granules in their cytoplasm.

Granulosa Cells

Primordial follicle cells that surround the ovum.

Graves' disease

An autoimmune disease in which thyroid stimulating immunoglobulins stimulate TSH receptors causing hyperthyroidism. Associated with bulging of the eyes (exophthalmos) and pretibial myxedema. *Also see hyperthyroidism and thyrotoxicosis.*

Gray Matter

The component of the central nervous system containing high concentrations of cell bodies, dendrites, and short non-myelinated fibers. Part of the sensory and motor neurons as well as interneurons are located in the gray matter. It also forms the cortex of the cerebrum and cerebral nuclei.

Growth Hormone

Also called *Somatotropic hormone,* it is secreted by the anterior pituitary and stimulates cell division, skeletal and soft tissue growth, and protein synthesis. Inadequate growth hormone production in childhood results in *dwarfism* while overproduction in adults results in *acromegaly. Also see gigantism.*

Gustation

Sense of taste. Taste disorders include: hypogeusia (decreased taste sensitivity), hypergeusia (increased taste sensitivity) and ageusia (lack of taste).

Gustducins

The particular types of G-proteins involved in the sense of taste; especially, of sweet and bitter tastes.

Gyrus

The elevated folds on the cerebral hemispheres caused by the infolding of the cortex (sulci). *Also see sulcus.*

H

H-Band

A component of muscle ultrastructure located at the center of the sarcomere; it consists of myosin fibers.

Hageman Factor

Factor XII of the clotting process.

Hagen-Poiseuille Equation

Originally applicable to flow of fluids through long cylindrical tubes; widely applicable in medicine to understand blood flow through vessels and gas flow through airways and anesthetic circuits. A version of the equation is shown as follows:

where
$$\text{Flow} = \frac{\Delta P \, r^4 \, \pi}{8 \, \eta \, L}$$

F= Flow, ΔP = pressure gradient, h = viscosity of blood, L = length of the vessel, and r = radius of the vessel. A doubling of the radius will increase flow 16 fold and a halving of the length will double the flow, all other factors remaining constant.

Jean Poiseuille (French physician) and G. Hagen (German engineer), 1846.

Hair Follicle Receptors

A type of sensory receptor that senses hair motion and direction.

Haldane Effect

The increased ability of reduced hemoglobin to carry carbon dioxide. Peripheral unloading of oxygen facilitates carbon dioxide loading from the tissues and the reverse phenomenon occurs in the lungs. *Also see Bohr effect and oxyhemoglobin dissociation curve.*

Haploid

Representing half the diploid number of chromosomes; characteristic of gametes (sperm and ova) which have only one set of chromosomes. Formation of a zygote restores the diploid number. *Also see Diploid.*

Hapten

A small molecule that causes antibody formation only when combined with larger "carrier" proteins that are immunogenic. Penicillin is an example.

Haptoglobin

A plasma protein that irreversibly binds free hemoglobin, preventing exposure of the kidneys to free hemoglobin. It is reduced in excessive hemolysis.

Hartnup's Disease	An unusual hereditary disease involving defective renal transport of neutral amino acids.
Haustration	A type of motility in the large intestine involving constrictive contractions of the muscle. These contractions divide the colon into compartments called haustra.
Haversian system	The basic structural unit of compact bone; consists of a haversian canal and its layers of bone. *After Clopton Havers- English physician and anatomist (1650 -1702).*
Hay Fever	A seasonal form of allergic rhinitis, characterized by inflammation of the nasal mucosa and conjunctiva (rhinitis and conjunctivitis); caused by pollen.
HCG (Human Chorionic Gonadotropin)	Hormone secreted by the embryo; main function is to prevent the normal involution of the corpus luteum at the end of the female sexual cycle. It is the basis for laboratory pregnancy testing. May be produced by other organs or by certain tumors e.g. trophoblastic disease. *Also see gonadotropins.*
Headache	Pain referred from stimuli arising from inside the cranium to the surface of the head. Pain may also arise from extra-cranial source e.g. nasal sinuses. Numerous types of headache have been described and a detailed history, physical examination, and testing may be required to ascertain its cause.
Hearing	The process of sound reception and perception.
Heart Block	An interruption of atrio-ventricular (AV) conduction; may range from a simple AV block to complete heart block. Ischemia of the conducting pathways is the most common cause. It also is seen after surgical correction of certain congenital heart defects in children. An artificial pacemaker is required in severe cases.
Heartburn	*See Pyrosis.*
Heart Failure	*See cardiogenic shock.*
Heart Murmur	An abnormal heart sound often caused by structural defects of the heart valves or septa. May occur with turbulent flow in the normal heart e.g. increased cardiac output states. This "functional" murmur is of no clinical significance.

Heart Rate

The number of heart beats per minute; approximately 70 beats per minute in normal adults, much higher in newborns and small children (usually >120/ min).

Heart Sounds

The sounds produced by closing of the heart valves. The first heart sound is due to closure of the mitral and tricuspid valves at the start of ventricular systole. Closure of the aortic and pulmonary valves at the end of ventricular systole produces the second heart sound.

Helicotrema

Tiny opening at the top of the cochlea through which the scala tympani and scala vestibule communicate.

Helper T Cells (CD4)

A type of T-cell (lymphocytes) that stimulates release of cytokines and other stimulatory molecules on exposure to an antigen; these cause helper T cells to divide and stimulates other immune cells to perform their functions. The Human immunodeficiency virus (HIV) infects these cells leading to Acquired immune deficiency syndrome (AIDS).

Hematocrit

The percentage of a blood sample that is made up of red blood cells. Also called packed cell volume (PCV).

Hematopoiesis

The process of blood cells formation. Impaired in chronic disease, renal disease and leukemia. Also impaired by chemotherapeutic agents. *Also see erythropoiesis.*

Heme

A red pigment containing one iron atom; combines with globin to form hemoglobin.

Hemoglobin

Red, iron-containing pigment formed by the combination of heme pigment and the protein globin present in red blood cells. It combines with and transports oxygen and (to a lesser degree) carbon dioxide. It is also a weak buffer within red blood cells.

Hemophilia

An inherited, X-linked, bleeding disorder; results from factor VIII deficiency (Hemophilia A) or factor IX deficiency (Hemophilia B or Christmas disease). Occurs almost exclusively in males and is associated with bleeding in the subcutaneous tissues, joints, and muscles.

Hemorrhage

Blood loss from vessels; in general, may be external or internal. If uncontrolled, hypovolemic shock will result. *Also see hypovolemic shock.*

Hemostasis

The various processes involved in the prevention and control of blood loss.

Henderson-Hasselbalch Equation

A formula that calculates the blood pH derived by a given ratio of bicarbonate to carbon dioxide concentrations. $P^H = P^K + Log [HCO3^-] / PaCO_2 (0.03)$ where P^K is the dissociation constant, which is 6.1 for the bicarbonate buffer system. The pH will be 7.40 as long as the ratio $[HCO3^-] / PaCO_2 (0.03)$ is 20:1. This is an important concept in the interpretation of arterial blood gases (ABG) in clinical practice. *Also see pH, acidosis, alkalosis, and buffers.*

Henry's Law

States that at a particular temperature, the amount of gas dissolved in a liquid is directly proportional to the partial pressure of the gas. Oxygen, carbon dioxide and nitrogen obey Henry's law. Decompression sickness is an example of the principle of Henry's law. *Also see decompression sickness.*

Heparin

A mucopolysaccharide abundant in the lungs and liver; it is an anticoagulant and also speeds the removal of fat particles from blood after a fatty meal. Used widely in clinical practice for its anticoagulant properties.

Hepatic Circulation

Blood flow to the liver; normally about 25% of the cardiac output. Liver blood flow arises from two sources: Hepatic portal veins and hepatic arteries. *Also see portal system.*

Hepatitis

Inflammation of the liver from a variety of causes:

Hepatitis A – caused by hepatitis A virus; is usually acquired from sewage-contaminated drinking water and sexual contact.

Hepatitis B – A DNA virus that is spread in the same way as HIV, the virus that causes AIDS.

Hepatitis C – caused by HCV; is usually acquired by contact with infected blood.

Hepatitis E – caused by HEV; common in developing countries. Also may be caused by other agents including autoimmune factors.

Hering-Breuer Reflex (Inflation reflex)

A reflex in which lung inflation stimulates stretch receptors resulting in apnea and augmentation of expiratory muscle contraction. Acts to limit inspiration. The reflex is strong in newborns but weak in adults

Hermaphrodite

An organism possessing male and female gonadal tissues. *Also see pseudohermaphrodite.*

Hexokinase

An enzyme that promotes the phosphorylation of glucose.

High-Density Lipoprotein (HDL)

A form in which cholesterol is carried in blood; it is presumed to be "good cholesterol" because it transports cholesterol to the liver for conversion to bile salts. It thus offers some protection against atherosclerosis and coronary artery disease. *Also see low-density lipoprotein (LDL).*

Higher Motor Neurons (Upper Motor Neurons)

Neuronal network forming part of the pyramidal and extrapyramidal systems; influence the activity of the lower motor neurons in the spinal cord.

Histamine

An autocoid produced from the amino acid histidine by decarboxylation. Pharmacologically, it acts on three subtypes of receptors:

H_1 receptors – mediate contraction of smooth muscles of ileum, uterus, bronchioles and blood vessels.

H_2 receptors – stimulate gastric secretion; mediate positive chronotropic and inotropic responses in the heart.

H_3 receptors – usually presynaptic and inhibit histamine release.

Histidine

An essential amino acid and the direct precursor of histamine; it is also important in purine synthesis

Histocompatibility Complex

Cell-surface antigens important for the function of T lymphocytes; located on all nucleated cells (except mature RBCs). *Also see HLA.*

Histone

Small, positively charged protein molecules associated with DNA; believed to repress genetic expression.

HLA (Human Leukocyte Antigen)

A group of tissue antigens located on the surface of white blood cells and play an important role in the body's immune system. Certain HLA types are believed to be associated with certain diseases. HLA typing is important in the area of transplantation medicine. Close HLA matching between the donor and recipient reduces the risk of rejection. *Also see Histocompatibility complex.*

HMG CoA
(β-hydroxy- β-methylglutaryl-CoA)

The precursor of cholesterol. HMG-CoA is converted to Mevalonic acid by the enzyme HMG-CoA reductase. This rate limiting step in cholesterol synthesis is the site of action of the "Statin" cholesterol-lowering drugs which inhibit the enzyme HMG-CoA reductase.

Homeostasis

Maintenance of the internal environment (milieu) within narrow limits; it is the basis of physiological regulatory mechanisms.

Homeotherm

An organism (e.g. mammals and birds) that maintains a constant body temperature independent of the environment.

Homologous Chromosomes

A term denoting similarly-constructed pairs of chromosomes in a diploid cell.

Homonymous Hemianopia

Loss of vision in the entire contralateral visual field due to a lesion of the entire optic tract radiation or visual cortex on one side.

Horizontal Cells

Provide lateral connections between the synaptic bodies of the rods and cones. Neural outputs are inhibitory thus ensuring adequate visual contrast into the CNS.

Hormone

A regulatory chemical messenger normally produced by endocrine glands; the secretions are released into the blood stream in low, physiologically-effective concentrations and transported to target cells where they influence metabolism or produce specific effects.

Horner's Syndrome

A syndrome resulting from interruption of the sympathetic innervation of the head and neck; characterized by: small appearing eyeball (enophthalmos), pupillary constriction, vasodilatation of the facial skin, absence of sweating on the affected side (anhidrosis) and nasal congestion. This is almost always seen with certain sympathetic blocks e.g. stellate ganglion block.

Humoral Immunity

Acquired immunity associated with antibody secretion in response to antigenic stimulation. *Also see B-Cell lymphocytes and plasma cells.*

Hunger

Craving for food; associated with increased appetite.

Huntington's disease

An autosomal dominant disorder of the basal ganglia resulting from a genetic defect on the short arm of chromosome 4; results in loss of GABAergic and cholinergic neurons in the striatum; characterized by progressive neuro-degeneration, chorea, and personality disorder.

Hyaline Membrane Disease

A disease caused by deficiency of surfactant, affecting premature infants or underdeveloped newborns; it is also called respiratory distress syndrome (RDS). Bovine surfactant is available for treating these infants and artificial ventilation is usually required. *Also see surfactant and pneumocytes.*

Hydrocephalus

Enlargement of the ventricles; commonly due to obstruction of CSF flow or impaired CSF resorption. Results in increased intracranial pressure that usually requires surgical intervention.

Hydrophilic

Denotes compounds or molecules that have an affinity for and readily dissolve in water. They usually possess strong polar groups that readily interact with water. *Also see lipohilic.*

Hydrophobic

Describes a type of molecule that does not dissolve in water because it is non-polar.

Hyperalgesia

Increased response to a painful stimulus. Perception of a non-painful stimulus as pain is called *allodynia*

Hyperbaric Oxygen

Also called *high-pressure oxygen;* Oxygen present at a pressure greater than one atmosphere. Hyperbaric oxygen has many therapeutic uses such as the treatment of carbon monoxide poisoning, certain clostridial infections, decompression sickness and difficult wound care. Exposure to excessive hyperbaric oxygen could result in oxygen toxicity.

Hypercapnia

Increased arterial partial pressure of CO_2 in the blood. Hypoventilation is a common cause.

Hyperemia

Increased blood flow to a part of the body. *Also see functional hyperemia.*

Hyperglycemia

A high blood glucose level. Seen in uncontrolled diabetes mellitus, stressful situations, and with certain medications.

Hyperkalemia

An abnormally high level of potassium in the blood. It has many causes and may cause EKG abnormalities.

Hyperopia

Also called long-sightedness or farsightedness. It occurs when the eyeball is abnormally short and rays from a distant object are brought into focus behind the retina. It is corrected by use of a biconvex lens. *Also see myopia and astigmatism.*

Hyperplasia

Increased growth of an organ caused by an increase in the number of cells. *Also see Hypertrophy.*

Hyperpnea

Abnormally deep or rapid breathing that occurs after exercise; proportional to the level of increase in muscle activity.

Hyperpolarization

An inhibitory state in excitable tissue in which there is an increase in the polarization (negativity) of the inside of a cell membrane with respect to the resting membrane potential.

Hyperpyrexia (Hyperthermia)

Extremely high fever; occurs particularly in children with certain infections. Malignant hyperthermia is a rare cause. *Also see fever and sarcoplasmic reticulum.*

Hypersensitivity

A state of an exaggerated immune response to a foreign body. There are 4 classic types: Type I (immediate, IgE-mediated), Type II (cytotoxic), Type III (immune complex) and Type IV (cell mediated) or delayed. Type V (autoimmune) has been described in certain literature. Also used to describe an allergic response to a drug or other foreign substance e.g. penicillin and latex. *Also see anaphylaxis, immediate and delayed hypersensitivity.*

Hypersomnia

A sleep disorder characterized by excessive sleepiness with difficulty staying awake.

Hypertension

Persistently high blood pressure; a systolic blood pressure greater than 140 mmHg or a diastolic blood pressure greater than 90 mmHg. In most cases, both systolic and diastolic blood pressures are elevated. Hypertension is classically divided into primary or essential (about 95% of cases) or secondary types. The two principal determinants of blood pressure are: the amount of blood pumped by the heart each minute – Cardiac output (CO) and the resistance to blood flow in the arteries – total peripheral resistance (TPR). Mathematically, BP = CO x TPR

Also see blood pressure.

Hyperthyroidism	A condition of thyroid gland over activity resulting in thyrotoxicosis. *See Grave's disease, thyrotoxicosis, and goiter.*
Hypertonic	Having a greater solute concentration and osmotic pressure relative to plasma.
Hypertrophy	A term denoting increased growth (enlargement) of a tissue or organ due to an increase in the cell size. *Also see hyperplasia.*
Hyperventilation	Increased rate and/or depth of breathing; results in decreased blood carbon dioxide tension. The cerebral vasoconstriction that results is the principle behind the use of this maneuver to lower intracranial pressure in certain situations.
Hypervolemia	An increase in circulating blood volume. Deliberate hypervolemia is used in hemodilution techniques for blood conservation during certain major surgical procedures.
Hypodermis	The layer of cells lying immediately beneath the epidermis.
Hypoglycemia	An inappropriately low blood glucose level for age. Symptoms include: shallow breathing, perspiration, tachycardia, pale skin, and anxiety (sympathetic stimulation).
Hypotension	A persistent decrease in the arterial blood pressure. If prolonged may result in end organ damage. The most common cause of hypotension in clinical practice is hypovolemia. Other causes are myocardial dysfunction/depression and a decrease in the systemic vascular resistance from certain drugs or neuraxial blocks (spinal or epidural). *Also see blood pressure.*
Hypothalamo-Hypophyseal Portal System	The vascular system that secretes and transports releasing and inhibiting hormones from the hypothalamus to the anterior pituitary.
Hypothalamo-Hypophyseal Tract	The neural pathway that transports antidiuretic hormone and oxytocin from the hypothalamus to the posterior pituitary.

Hypothalamus

The part of the brain located below the thalamus and above the pituitary gland. The hypothalamus regulates the body's internal environment and produces releasing factors that control the anterior pituitary.

Hypothermia

A decrease in body temperature below 36.0 °C. Associated with a decreased oxygen requirement. Accidental causes include environmental exposure, immersion, and certain drug overdoses. Deliberate hypothermia is utilized in certain surgical procedures (cardiac and neurosurgery) for organ protection.

Hypotonia

A decrease in muscle tone. Often a sign of an underlying neurological, muscle, neuromuscular junction, metabolic, or mitochondrial disease.

Hypovolemic Shock

Shock due to an inadequate intravascular volume (preload). Usually occurs when blood volume has been reduced by 30-40 %. Hemorrhage is a leading cause. Also seen in severe vomiting and diarrhea, burns, severe infections, and excessive diuresis. *Also see shock, preload, and renal failure.*

Hypoxemia

A decrease in blood arterial oxygen tension. Causes include: hypoventilation, decreased inspired oxygen tension as in high altitude, certain lung diseases and ventilation/perfusion mismatch.

Hypoxia

A decreased oxygen supply to the tissues. There are four types:

- *Hypoxic hypoxia*: (or arterial hypoxemia) – associated with low alveolar PO_2, due to low PO_2 in inspired air or hypoventilation
- *Anemic hypoxia*: - associated with low or abnormal hemoglobins, due to anemia, CO poisoning or hemoglobinopathies
- *Stagnant hypoxia*: - associated with inadequate blood flow to tissues, due to cardiac failure or local ischemia
- *Cytotoxic hypoxia*: In the true sense, is not a lack of supply but a failure of oxygen utilization as in cyanide poisoning.

I

I- Band	A component of muscle ultrastructure containing actin filaments; isotropic to polarized light.
Ifosfamide	A chemotherapeutic agent used in the treatment of certain types of cancer. It inhibits DNA synthesis by alkylating guanine.
Ileogastric Reflex	A reflex initiated by distension of the ileum; results in decreased gastric motility. *Also see gastroileal reflex.*
Ilium	The superior portion of the hip bone (innominate bone). The other bones are the ischium and pubis.
Immediate Hypersensitivity	An allergic response mediated by IgE class of antibodies; results in the release of histamine and related compounds from cells (mast cells and basophils) when antigens combine with specific IgE antibodies. It is the classic anaphylactic response (type I). *Also see hypersensitivity reactions and anaphylaxis.*
Immune cytolysis	Antibody-mediated cell lysis. Participation of complement is also involved.
Immunity	The capacity of the human body to resist most types of foreign bodies or toxins that can cause tissue or organ damage.
Immunization	A strategy for increasing a person's resistance to pathogens. Active immunity is produced by injection of antigens that stimulate the development of clones of specific B or T lymphocytes. In passive immunity, a non-immune individual is given prepared antibodies by injection of antibodies or sensitized immune cells made by immune individuals.
Immunoassay	Laboratory or clinical technique using specific bonding between an antigen and its homologous antibody to identify and quantify a substance in a sample.
Immunoblast	A type of cell produced by transformation of T lymphocytes following antigen stimulation; the resulting T cells have specificity against the stimulating antigen.
Immunodeficiency	A disorder in which there is a deficiency of the immunological response to infections. Seen in certain

primary immunodeficiency syndromes and AIDS (Acquired immune deficiency syndrome).

Immunoglobulins

Globular plasma proteins that have antibody functions, providing humoral immunity. They are classified as: IgM, IgG, IgE, IgD and IgA. IgG is the most abundant, constituting about 75% of immunoglobulins in human serum. Intravenous immune globulin (IVIG) contains pooled IgG and has wide therapeutic application in clinical practice. *Also see gamma globulin and immunotherapy.*

Immunosuppression

Prevention or attenuation of the immune response; it can be caused by drugs or radiation. It can also be medically induced to control autoimmune diseases and prevent transplant or graft rejection.

Immunosurveillance

The cell-mediated function of the immune system to recognize and attack malignant cells that produce antigens not recognized as "self."

Immunotherapy

A general term for the use of various immune modulation methods to treat various diseases. Includes immunization, immunosuppression, immune augmentation, and the treatment of certain cancers using cytokines. *Also see immunoglobulins.*

Implantation

The process by which the embryo attaches itself to and penetrates the lining of the uterus (endometrium).

Incus

The middle of the three ossicles of the ear. Responsible for conduction of vibrations from the tympanic membrane to the inner ear.

In vitro

Taking place outside the body or in an artificial environment. In vitro fertilization (test tube baby) is a good example.

In vivo

Occurring within the body.

Infarct

An area of necrotic tissue resulting from obstruction of blood flow or inadequate blood flow (ischemia). Myocardial infarction is a classic example. *Also see ischemia.*

Infertility

Absence of conception despite frequent sexual intercourse. Most common causes are: blocked fallopian tubes, endometriosis and a low sperm count or presence of a large proportion of abnormal spermatozoa.

Inflammatory Response

See triple response.

Inhibin

A glycoprotein circulating in plasma; secreted by the seminiferous tubules of the testes. It specifically exerts negative feedback control of the secretion of follicle-stimulating hormone from the anterior pituitary.

Inositol 1, 4, 5-Triphosphate (IP$_3$)

A second messenger in signal transduction pathways; produced by the cell membrane of a target cell in response to the action of a hormone. IP$_3$ binds to specific ligand-gated Ca^{2+} channels in the endoplasmic reticulum and induces Ca^{2+} release.

Inspiratory Reserve Volume (IRV)

The total volume of air that can be inhaled above the normal tidal volume following a maximal inspiratory effort. It is about 3 Liters in an adult male. The IRV together with the tidal volume (TV) and the expiratory reserve volume (ERV) constitute the forced vital capacity (FVC).

Insulin

A naturally-occurring polypeptide hormone secreted by the beta cells of the islets of Langerhans in the pancreas. Insulin lowers blood glucose by promoting the cellular uptake of blood glucose and the conversion of glucose to glycogen by the liver and skeletal muscles. Insulin deficiency produces hyperglycemia and diabetes mellitus. Insulin therapy is the mainstay of anti-diabetic treatment, especially type I diabetes.

Insulin-Like Growth Factors (IGFs)

Also called *somatomedins*; exist in two forms: IGF-1 and IGF-2; circulating IGFs are produced primarily in the liver under the influence of growth hormone.

Integration

Neuronal summation of excitatory and inhibitory signals.

Intercalated Disks

Specialized structures that bind cardiac muscle cells together in an end to end fashion; they represent areas of low electrical resistance.

Interferons

Species-specific proteins (cytokines) produced by virus-infected cells; they increase the resistance of non-infected cells. They have anti-proliferative and immune modulation effects and are used in the treatment of many conditions such as: Hepatitis C infection, certain leukemias, laryngeal papillomatosis, hemangiomas, AIDS-related Kaposi sarcoma and malignant melanoma.

Interleukin-2 (IL-2)

A lymphokine secreted by T-cells in response to antigens; it is used in immunotherapy to treat certain cancers because of its ability to stimulate the immune system to kill tumor cells and decrease tumor blood flow.

Intermediate Filaments (IFs)

One of three different elements (including actin microfilaments and tubulin microtubules) that constitutes the network of fibrous proteins crossing throughout the cytoskeleton and the nuclear boundary of animal cells. In muscles cells, their diameters range from 8-10 nm, intermediate between those of thin filaments (actin, 6 nm) and thick filaments (myosin, 15 nm). They function as cellular stress absorbers and play a role in cell plasticity. The main IF protein in mature skeletal and cardiac muscle is *desmin*. *Also see desmin, actin, myosin, thin and thick filaments.*

Interneuron

A neuron that conveys information between neurons in the CNS.

Internodal fibers

See cardiac conducting system.

Interstitial Cells (*of Leydig*)

Located in the interstices between the seminiferous tubules; present in large numbers in adult males and secrete testosterone and other androgenic hormones.

Interstitial Space

The space between capillaries, between capillaries and alveoli vessels, and between alveoli.

Intrafusal Fibers

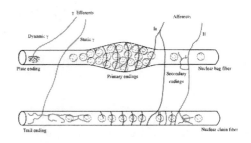

Specialized muscle spindle fibers that are innervated by γ-motor neurons and encapsulated to form muscle spindle organs, essentially muscle stretch receptors. The two types of intrafusal fibers are: Nuclear bag and nuclear chain. The static and dynamic gamma-motor neurons regulate the sensitivity of the intrafusal muscle fibers. *Also see extrafusal fibers, nuclear bag fibers, and nuclear chain fibers*

Intrapleural Space

Space between the parietal pleura (membrane lining the chest cavity) and the visceral pleura (membrane lining the lungs); it contains a thin layer of fluid (20-25 mL in the average adult) which provides lubrication between them. Intrapleural analgesia is a useful technique for pain control for upper abdominal and thoracic surgery, cancer pain, and pain from multiple rib fractures. *Also see pleural cavity and pneumothorax.*

Intrapulmonary Space

The space within the air sacs and airways of the lungs.

Intrinsic Factor

A glycoprotein secreted by gastric parietal cells; needed for vitamin B12 absorption. In the absence of intrinsic factor, vitamin B12 is not absorbed, resulting in *pernicious anemia*.

Intron

A segment of a gene located between coding regions (exons); it does not code for proteins.

Inulin

A fructose polysaccharide produced from rhizomes of certain plants; inulin clearance is used in renal function tests to assess glomerular filtration rate since it is freely filtered across the glomerulus – it is neither secreted nor reabsorbed. *Also see renal clearance and glomerular filtration rate.*

Iodothyronines

Secretory products of the thyroid gland derived from the coupling of two iodinated tyrosine molecules.

Ion

An atom or group of atoms having a net electric charge resulting from the loss or gain of electrons.

Ion Channels

Membrane protein structures that permit movement of small ions across the membrane. Stimuli for opening of ion channels include: neurotransmitter (receptor gated), membrane potential change (voltage-gated), calcium ions (calcium gated) and G-proteins.

IP_3

See inositol 1,4,5,-triphosphate.

Ipsilateral

On the same side (as opposed to contralateral).

IPSP (Inhibitory postsynaptic potential)

A hyperpolarizing current on the postsynaptic neuronal membrane induced by the interaction between an inhibitory neurotransmitter from the presynaptic neuron and receptors on the postsynaptic neuronal membrane. IPSPs reduce the excitability of the postsynaptic membrane by making it difficult to generate action potentials.

Iron-Deficiency Anemia

A type of anemia characterized by smaller than normal (microcytic) and hypochromic red blood cells. *Also see anemia.*

Ischemia

Inadequate blood flow to an organ or structure; usually caused by obstruction or constriction of the blood vessel supplying the organ or structure. Examples are myocardial or cerebral ischemia. *Also see infarct.*

Islets Of Langerhans	Clusters of cells within the pancreas containing: alpha cells (which secrete glucagon), beta cells (which secrete insulin) and delta cells (which secrete somatostatin). Also called pancreatic islets.
Isometric Contraction	A type of muscle contraction in which the muscle length remains constant but muscle tension increases. Weight-lifting is a good example.
Isoproterenol	A non-selective β-adrenergic agonist that is used for the treatment of certain heart blocks and pulmonary hypertension. Produces bronchodilation but is rarely used for asthma treatment because of its non-selectivity.
Isosorbide dinitrate	A coronary and peripheral vasodilator commonly used to treat and prevent angina pectoris and coronary insufficiency. Isosorbide-5-mononitrate is an active metabolite of the parent compound. *Also see angina pectoris.*
Isotonic Contraction	A type of muscle contraction in which the muscle contracts and shortens while tension remains constant. An example of isotonic contraction is flexing the biceps muscle.
Isotonic Solution	A solution having equal amounts of dissolved solutes within and outside of the cell.
Isovolumic Contraction	A period of constant ventricular volume during the cardiac cycle; it corresponds to the time interval between the start of ventricular systole and the opening of the aortic and pulmonary valves.
Isovolumic Relaxation	The time interval during the cardiac cycle between closure of the pulmonary and aortic valves and opening of the atrioventricular (AV) valves; ventricular pressure falls drastically but ventricular volume remains constant.

J

J-receptors (Juxta-capillary receptors)

Receptors present in alveolar walls and in close proximity to the capillaries; presumed to play a role in dyspnea and shallow breathing in patients with left ventricular heart failure as well as in patients with interstitial lung disease.

Jaundice

The presence of increased levels of bilirubin in the blood. It is associated with yellow coloration of the skin and mucous membranes. *Also see bilirubin and Kernicterus.*

Jaw Jerk

A stretch reflex in which tapping the chin, with the mouth partially open and the jaw supported, stretches the masseter muscles causing contraction and jerking of the jaw.

Jejunum

A region of the small intestine important for absorption, particularly of ions.

Jugular Venous Pressure (JVP)

The indirectly observed pressure over the venous system. Careful observation of the different wave forms could yield important diagnostic clues.

Junctional Complexes

Complex multi-receptor-like structures that join adjacent epithelial cells together; they function in the regulation of cell differentiation and growth.

Juxtaglomerular Apparatus

A renal structure consisting of the glomerular afferent and efferent arterioles and specialized cells called the macula densa. The juxtaglomerular cells, located in the afferent arterioles of the glomerulus, are the site of release of the enzyme renin. *Also see renin.*

K

Kalidin

See kallikrein.

Kallikrein

A proteolytic enzyme found in blood and tissue fluids in an inactive form; upon activation, it acts on alpha$_2$-globulin to release *kalidin* (a kinin) that is subsequently converted into the vasodilator bradykinin. *Also see bradykinin.*

Kaposi's sarcoma

An unusual cancer of blood vessels that produces reddish-purple, coin-sized lesions and spots on the skin and mucus membranes. It is caused by human herpes virus 8 (HHV8). Previously very rare and found mostly in organ transplant patients and elderly men of Eastern European or Mediterranean origin and African men, it is now mostly seen in HIV/AIDS patients. It is the most common cancer in AIDS patients. *Named after Dr. Moritz Kaposi (Hungarian dermatologist) who first described it in 1872.*

Karyotype

Paired arrangement, in a fixed order, of all the chromosomes within a cell.

Keratin

Major protein component of the outer layer of the epidermis, hair and nails.

Kernicterus

Encephalopathy resulting from deposition of unconjugated bilirubin in the brain cells of severely jaundiced newborns. Erythroblastosis fetalis is a major risk factor for kernicterus. Lethal in extreme cases and neurological deficits are usually inevitable in those who survive. Severe hyperbilirubinemia is treated by phototherapy and exchange blood transfusion (EBT). *Also see bilirubin and jaundice.*

Ketoacidosis

Metabolic acidosis resulting from the excessive production of ketone bodies as in diabetic ketoacidosis.

Ketogenesis

The process of ketone bodies production.

Ketone Bodies

Substances consisting of acetone, acetoacetic acid, and β-hydroxybutyric acid; they are produced by hepatocytes from fatty acids, via acetyl CoA. Skeletal muscles oxidize ketone bodies for energy.

Ketonuria

Presence of ketone bodies in the urine as seen in diabetic ketoacidosis.

Ketosis	Excessively high blood concentration of ketone bodies. It is associated with a rapid breakdown of fat, e.g. during dieting or in uncontrolled diabetes mellitus.
Kidney failure	*See renal failure.*
Killer Cells	Cytotoxic T cells capable of killing microorganisms and sometimes, even the body's own cells.
Kilocalorie	The amount of heat required to raise the temperature of 1 kilogram of water by 1°C.
Kinesiology	The study of the interactions of different muscle groups.
Kininogens	Plasma protein precursors of the local vasodilators bradykinin and kalidin.
Kinocilium	A very large cilium located on the hair cells of the vestibular apparatus; aids impulse transmission.
Klinefelter's Syndrome	A syndrome produced in males with a 47, XXY karyotype. Associated with hypogonadism, infertility and mental retardation (in some patients). May also have 48, XXXY karyotype.
Kluver-Bucy Syndrome	Results from bilateral temporal lobe lesions; it is characterized by decreased emotions, hypersexuality, attention to irrelevant stimuli and visual agnosia.
Knee Jerk	A stretch reflex initiated by striking the patellar ligament with a rubber mallet.
Knockout Mice	Strains of mice that have been genetically-engineered to lack a specific gene or genes; they are therefore unable to express the protein coded for by that gene. This provides researchers information about what that gene normally does and what a lack or mutation of the specific gene could cause. Knockout mice have been used as animal models to study cancers, obesity, aging, and substance abuse. *Also see p53 and gene therapy.*
Korotkoff Sounds	Sounds heard by auscultation during blood pressure measurement; caused by blood jetting through the partially-occluded vessel. *Also see auscultatory blood pressure measurement.*
Krebs cycle	Also called citric acid cycle; a cyclical metabolic pathway in the mitochondrial matrix by which acetyl groups

are broken down to CO_2 and H_2O in aerobic cellular respiration with release of ATP.

Krause End Bulbs Pressure-sensitive proprioceptors.

Kupffer Cells Phagocytic cells (macrophages) lining the sinusoids of the liver; they are a part of the reticuloendothelial system.

Kwashiorkor (Protein Calorie Malnutrition) A protein deficiency syndrome, associated with growth retardation, generalized edema, lethargy and immunodeficiency. Common in under-developed countries especially in war-torn areas. The term means *"the displaced or deposed child"* in the Ga language of Ghana, West Africa. *Also see Marasmus.*

Kyphosis An abnormal posterior curvature of the vertebral column that results in a hunchback (kyphos).

L

L-type Channels	Type of Ca^{2+} channels in which activation involves passage of long-lasting current; they constitute the predominant types of Ca^{2+} channels in the heart. The channels are blocked by Ca^{2+} channel blockers such as Nifedipine, Verapamil, and Diltiazem. *Also see calcium channel blockers and T-type channels.*
Lacis Cells	Mesanglial cells located outside the glomerulus between the afferent and efferent arterioles. They have a phagocytic function and are a part of the juxtaglomerular apparatus. *Also see juxtaglomerular apparatus.*
Lacrimal Glands	Glands in the eye responsible for tear secretion.
Lactate Threshold	Denotes the intensity of exercise; the average lactate threshold is achieved when exercise is performed at 50% to 70% of the maximal oxygen uptake (aerobic capacity).
Lactose Intolerance	The condition of impaired or lack of activity of lactase enzyme; this results in inability to digest lactose. Lactose is the predominant sugar in milk. Lactase enzyme is available in tablet and liquid forms for lactose intolerant individuals. A variety of lactose-free and lactose-reduced dairy products are also widely available.
Laplace's law	States that the stress in the vessel wall produced by the transmural pressure (P) in a distensible hollow object is proportional to the wall tension (T) and inversely proportional to the radius (R). Mathematically, $P = T/R$ for a cylinder and $P = 2T/R$ for a sphere. This important principle has many applications:

- Surfactant reduces surface tension in the alveoli as the radius decreases during expiration thus preventing collapse from the increased transmural pressure.
- The dilated heart in *heart failure* patients would need to develop more tension to produce a given intraventricular pressure hence the benefit of preload reduction.

Larynx	A musculo-cartilaginous structure located between the pharynx and the trachea; it acts as a valve controlling

entrance into the trachea and functions as a voice box for phonation. It is composed of one bone (hyoid), three single cartilages and three paired cartilages held together by ligaments and muscles. A thorough understanding of the anatomy and physiology of the larynx is essential for all health care workers especially those in the acute care setting. Direct visualization of the larynx (laryngoscopy) is performed to facilitate endotracheal intubation and diagnose various diseases of the airway.

Lateral Inhibition

Enhanced contrast in the perception of sensory signals. Input from those receptors that are most greatly stimulated is enhanced while input from other receptors is decreased. Enhanced transmission of visual patterns into the central nervous system is an example of this phenomenon

Length-Tension Relationship

Describes the phenomenon whereby the strength of a muscle's contraction depends on the initial length of the muscle fibers under resting condition. Maintenance of the muscle length is by way of reflex contraction induced by passive stretch. The strength of muscle contraction is reduced when the muscle is shorter or longer than its normal length.

Lens

Clear, membrane-like structure found in the eye; it is responsible for bringing objects into focus on the retina.

Leptin

A protein hormone secreted by adipose tissue; it acts on the hypothalamus to signal satiety and reduce appetite. Leptin is believed to cross the blood brain barrier via receptors on endothelial cells and produces two effects: activation of catabolic circuits and repression of anabolic circuits.

Leukemia

A cancer of blood-forming tissues; characterized by infiltration of the bone marrow with large numbers of immature white blood cells, thus impairing development of all cell lines. Traditionally classified as acute or chronic, leukemias are the most common childhood cancers, accounting for about 30% of all childhood malignancies. Leukemias are also common in adults.

Leukocytes

Also called white blood cells; provide defense for the body. Sites of formation include: bone marrow (granulocytes, monocytes and some lymphocytes) and lymph tissue (lymphocytes and plasma cells). The percentages of the different types of leucocytes are: Neutrophils, 62%, eosinophils 2.3%, basophils 0.4%, monocytes 5.3%, and lymphocytes 30%.

Leukopenia

A reduction in the number of leukocytes (white blood cells) in the blood below 5×10^9 per liter. The absolute neutrophil count (ANC) is a measure of the actual neutrophil granulocytes number in the circulation. It is derived by multiplying the percentage of neutrophils and bands by the WBC. A value less than 1500 cells/μL is defined as neutropenia and a value less than 500 is severe neutropenia. The common causes are infections (HIV-AIDS), drug-induced, marrow replacement (leukemias and solid tumors), chemotherapy and malnutrition.

Leukotrienes

Eicosanoids that are closely related to prostaglandins; leukotrienes are formed from arachidonic acid by the action of 5-lipoxygenase. They were formerly called slow-reacting substance of anaphylaxis (SRS-A). Various types of leukotrienes (LTB_4, LTC_4, LTD_4 and LTE_4) have been identified. They are potent inflammatory mediators and LTC_4, LTD_4 and LTE_4 are potent bronchoconstrictors. Montelukast (Singulair) and Zafirlukast (Accolate®) are relatively new selective leukotriene D4-receptor antagonists used in the treatment of asthma. *Also see asthma, eicosanoids, non-steroidal antiinflamatory drugs and cyclooxygenase.*

Leydig Cells

See Interstitial cells.

Ligament

Fibrous band of dense regular connective tissue that joins bone to bone at joints; it also serves to strengthen joints.

Ligand

Refers to:

(i) A radioactively–labeled drug employed in receptor binding studies.

(ii) A structural group on an endogenous or exogenous biological substance involved in receptor binding.

Light Adaptation

A rapid process involving reduction in photoreceptor sensitivity upon entry into a bright room; due to reduction in the amount of rhodopsin. Light adaptation occurs within seconds and favors cone vision.

Limb Leads (Standard)

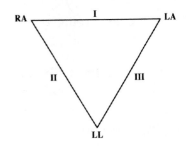

Electrocardiographic lead system devised by Einthoven in which the vector sum of all the heart's electrical activity at any given moment is presumed to lie in the center of an imaginary triangle formed by the left and right shoulders and the left leg. There are three standard limb leads: I, II and III. *Also see Einthoven's triangle.*

Limbic System

Represents a network of fiber tracts and nuclei forming the medial portions of the cerebral hemispheres, subcortical nuclei and the diencephalon; it contains the hippocampus and the amygdala. Essential for memory, learning, and emotions.

Lipases

Fat- digesting enzymes.

Lipid

A non-polar organic molecule, insoluble in water; notably triglycerides, steroids, and phospholipids.

Lipogenesis

The process of formation of fat or triglycerides.

Lipolysis

The hydrolysis of triglycerides into free fatty acids and glycerol.

Lipophilic

Non-polar molecules; soluble in lipids; e.g. steroid and thyroid hormones and the lipid-soluble vitamins. *Also see hydrophilic.*

Lipoproteins

Organic compound consisting of both protein and lipids. Lipoproteins constitute the principal means by which lipids are transported in blood. The various types of lipoproteins are:

- Chylomicrons - transport fat from the intestines to the liver and to adipose tissue.
- Very low density lipoproteins (VLDL) - transport freshly-synthesized triacylglycerol from the liver to adipose tissue
- Intermediate density lipoproteins (IDL) - are intermediate between VLDL and LDL. Usually present in trace amount in blood
- Low density lipoproteins (LDL) - called "bad cholesterol" lipoprotein because it transports cholesterol from the liver to cells. LDLs are believed to contribute to artherosclerosis.

- High density lipoproteins (HDL) - called "good cholesterol" lipoprotein - transport cholesterol from the tissues back to the liver.

Hypercholesterolemia is an important risk factor for the development of coronary artery disease. *Also see HMG-CoA and high-density lipoprotein (HDL).*

Lipostatic Theory   *See Food Intake.*

Lithiasis   Pathological condition characterized by the formation of stones (calculi) in internal organs; e.g. biliary or urinary calculi. Cholelithiasis (gall stones) and nephrolithiasis (kidney stone) are common causes of abdominal pain and other symptoms and often require surgical intervention.

Liver   A vital organ with many important functions including: Metabolism, production and secretion of bile, protein synthesis, glycogen storage and detoxification of harmful substances.

Long-Term Potentiation   Enhanced synaptic efficacy commonly observed in repetitive activation of an afferent pathway to the hippocampus; appears to involve both pre- and post-synaptic events and is mediated by some neurotransmitters e.g. excitatory amino acids (EAAs).

Loop of Henle   Part of the nephron consisting of a descending and an ascending limb; located between the proximal and the distal convoluted tubule; it is important for water reabsorption by the countercurrent mechanism.

Low-Density Lipoproteins (LDL)   *See lipoproteins and high-density lipoprotein (HDL).*

Lower Esophageal Sphincter (LES)   Also called *gastro-esophageal sphincter*. Failure of the LES to relax results in impairment of swallowing (achalasia). An absent or decreased intra-abdominal esophagus causes LES malfunction and is a common cause of gastro-esophageal reflux disease (GERD). Both of these conditions usually require surgical correction, the former by esophageal dilatation or a Heller myotomy and the latter by fundoplication. *Also see upper esophageal sphincter.*

Lower Motor Neuron (LMN)   An efferent neuron with its cell body in the gray matter of the spinal cord; contributes axons to peripheral nerves and innervates muscles and glands and is under the control of the upper motor neurons. *Also see upper motor neuron and motor neuron disease.*

Lung Surfactant

Lipoproteins (dipamitoyl phosphatidyl choline) produced by type II alveolar cells into the alveoli. Appears in the late stages of fetal development and serves to lower surface tension thus preventing alveolar collapse at low lung volumes. Surfactant deficiency in premature infants causes hyaline membrane disease (respiratory distress syndrome) of the newborn. Use of bovine or synthetic surfactant is now an established treatment for this condition.

Lupus Erythematosus (systemic)

A chronic inflammatory autoimmune disease of unknown etiology: characterized by generalized involvement of the joints, skin, muscles, lungs, kidneys, and other organs. Anti-nuclear antibodies (ANA) and Anti-DNA antibodies are commonly found in the sera of patients with Lupus. It is 8 times more common in women and may also occur in children.

Luteinizing Hormone (LH)

A glycoprotein gonadotropic hormone secreted by the anterior pituitary. In females, it stimulates development of the corpus luteum while in males, it stimulates production of testosterone.

Luteolysis

Regression of the corpus luteum in the absence of fertilization and pregnancy; associated with necrosis of the endocrine cells and invasion by leukocytes, macrophages and fibroblasts.

Lymph

A fluid derived from tissue fluid; it is carried in lymphatic vessels.

Lymphatic System

A system made up of lymphatic vessels and lymphoid organs.

Lymphocyte

Mononuclear leukocyte that functions in the development of humoral (B lymphocytes) and cell-mediated (T lymphocytes) immunity. *Also see humoral immunity.*

Lymphokines

Chemicals released from T cells that contribute to cell-mediated immunity.

Lysine

An essential amino acid; lysine deficiency can lead to a deficiency in niacin (a B vitamin), resulting in *pellagra*.

Lysoferrin   Bactericidal agent contained in lysosomes; binds iron and other metals necessary for bacterial growth.

Lysosomes   Membrane-bound organelles containing the digestive enzymes of a cell.

M

M Gate

Also called *Activation Gate*: located in fast Na$^+$ channels in the membrane of excitable cells; it causes the channels to open when resting membrane potential becomes less negative.

Macromolecule

A large molecule consisting of structural subunits that are linked. Proteins, starches and nucleic acids are examples.

Macrophage

Type of white blood cells (leukocytes) found mainly in the lymph and connective tissues in all vertebrates. Macrophages eliminate bacteria and other microorganisms by phagocytosis and thus contribute to both specific and nonspecific immunity.

Macula

See macula lutea.

Macula Densa

A short segment of the thick ascending limb of the nephron that is in contact with the afferent arteriole. It senses an increased flow of filtrate and causes the afferent arterioles to constrict, thus lowering glomerular filtration rate.

Macula Lutea

A small, sensitive, and yellowish central area in the retina. It contains the fovea centralis and is very rich in cones. It is the area with the highest visual acuity and is responsible for detailed central vision such as reading or watching television. Macula degeneration is a major cause of visual deterioration in individuals older than 50 years. *Also see fovea centralis.*

Macula Sacculi /Utriculi

Sensory epithelia of the otolith organs of the ear. *Also see otolith organ.*

Malignant

Refers to a life-threatening disease process. A rapidly progressing condition.

Malleus

One of the three ossicles of the ear; conducts sound vibrations from the tympanic membrane to the inner ear.

Mammary Glands

The secretory tissues of the breasts; consist of elongated slender ducts.

Marasmus

Severe malnutrition due to an inadequate caloric intake

with total inanition (severe weakness and emaciation) in a young child. *Also see Kwashiorkor.*

Mass Movements

A wave of contraction occurring in the colon at a rate of 1-3 times daily.

Mast Cells

Found throughout extravascular tissues and containing many granules; they release histamine on stimulation. Granules also contain heparin and several proteases. *Also see anaphylaxis.*

Mastication

See chewing.

Mean Arterial Pressure (MAP)

The "average" arterial pressure during a cardiac cycle. Mathematically, mean arterial pressure = diastolic pressure + 1/3 pulse pressure. Pulse pressure is: systolic BP – Diastolic BP. It is not a true average because of the difference in diastolic and systolic times. *Also see pulse pressure.*

Mean Circulatory Pressure

An equilibrium pressure in the circulatory system in the absence of flow.

Mean Electrical Axis

The net direction of electrical potential during ventricular depolarization. In normal ventricles the value is about 60 degrees. *Also see electrical axis.*

Mechanical Allodynia

A condition in which activation of mechanoreceptors causes pain. *Also see hyperalgesia*

Mechanoreceptor

A sensory receptor that is mechanically stimulated; it is important for tactile and position senses. Examples are pressure receptors, stretch receptors and hair cells. *Also see Meissner's corpuscles.*

Medulla Oblongata

The region of the brain located between the spinal cord and the pons; it contains vital neural centers for the regulation of the respiratory and the cardiovascular systems.

Megakaryocyte

Large bone marrow cells that are the precursors of platelets.

Meiosis

A type of cell division that occurs in the process of gamete production in the gonads; it results in four daughter cells containing the haploid number of 23 chromosomes. It requires two cell divisions – meiosis I and meiosis II. *Also see mitosis and telophase.*

Meissner's Corpuscles

Rapidly-adapting cutaneous mechanoreceptors. *Also see mechanoreceptors.*

Meissner's Plexus

Also called *submucosal plexus*; a network of nerve cells located in the submucosa of the wall of the gastrointestinal tract.

Melanin

A dark pigment responsible for the normal coloration of the hair, skin and eyes. It is also present in the substantia nigra (brain) and in certain tumors (melanomas).

Melanocytes

Cells located at the border between the dermis and epidermis; they produce the dark pigment, melanin.

Melanocyte-Stimulating Hormone (MSH)

Secreted by the anterior pituitary gland; stimulates melanin production by melanocytes.

Melatonin (5-methoxy-N-acetyltryptamine)

A hormone derived from serotonin and secreted by pinealocytes in the pineal gland; it plays a role in the circadian rhythm. Melatonin levels are high at night (as we get sleepy) and low during the day. Melatonin acts as an endocrine hormone (produced by the pineal gland) or paracrine hormone (produced by the retina and the GI tract). Melatonin supplements are available for use as a sleeping aid and in the treatment of symptoms of jet lag.

Membrane Potential

The potential difference that exists between the inside and outside of the cell membrane due to the relative distribution of charged particles across the membrane. It exists in all cells but is of particular importance in excitable cells (cells capable of self-generation of electrochemical impulses at their membranes such as nerve and muscle cells). In the non-stimulated state, the membrane potential is called *resting potential* and the lining of the membrane interior is negatively charged. It ranges from –70 mV to –90 mV.

Membranous Labyrinth

The functional part of the vestibular apparatus; it is composed of the cochlea, three semicircular ducts, the utricle and the saccule. *Also see vestibular system.*

Memory

Ability to hold a thought in mind or to recall events from the past. It is comparable to the storage and retrieval system of a computer. There are two types of memory: *short-term* and *long-term*. The brain areas responsible for the memory process include: the hippocampus, amygdala and the mammillary bodies.

Menarche

The first menstrual period; usually occurs during puberty.

Ménière's disease

A disorder of the inner ear characterized by vestibular nystagmus, vertigo and "ringing in the ears" (tinnitus). *Also see tinnitus and vertigo.*

Menopause

The period of a woman's life when the ovarian and uterine cycles terminate; usually occurs at about age 50.

Menstrual Cycle

The cyclic production of estrogen and progesterone and the changes in the endometrium that culminates in the desquamation of the endometrium. It is regulated by the hypothalamus through the anterior pituitary gland.

Menstruation

Periodic shedding of blood cells from the uterine lining; occurs about every 28 days.

MEPP

See miniature end plate potential.

Meromyosin

A subunit of the myosin molecule; it consists of two types: heavy and light meromyosin.

Mesencephalon

The midbrain; functions includes: control of eye movement, motor control, and acoustic relay.

Mesenchyme

A component of embryonic mesoderm that gives rise to connective tissue, bone, cartilage and the circulatory and lymphatic systems.

Mesoderm

The middle germ layer of embryonic tissue that gives rise to connective tissue, the circulatory system, muscles and the adrenal cortex.

Mesothelioma

A rare form of malignant cancer of the pleura, but may also affect the peritoneum and the pericardium. It is usually associated with asbestos exposure.

Mesothelium

A layer of flat cells derived from the mesoderm; it lines the body cavity in embryonic life and forms the simple epithelium in adult life.

Messenger RNA (mRNA)

A type of RNA that contains the code for the production of a particular protein.

Metabolic Acidosis

Increased hydrogen ion concentration in arterial blood ($\downarrow$pH inappropriate for arterial CO_2 level); due to increased non-volatile acids or a decreased amount of bicarbonate. Common causes include ketoacidosis, lactic acidosis, salicylate or ethylene glycol poisoning, renal failure, renal tubular acidosis, diarrhea, and gastrointestinal, biliary or pancreatic fistulae. *Also see respiratory acidosis.*

Metabolic Alkalosis
Decreased hydrogen ion concentration in arterial blood (↑pH inappropriate for arterial CO_2 level); due to acid loss as in prolonged vomiting and renal acid loss or excess base ingestion or administration. *Also see respiratory alkalosis.*

Metabolic Breathing
Concerned with oxygen delivery to the mitochondria as well as acid-base balance arising from the effect of breathing on blood CO_2.

Metabolism
All of the chemical processes occurring within a cell; it includes anabolism (energy storage) and catabolism (energy liberation).

Metarhodopsin
A breakdown product of the photochemical, rhodopsin.

Metastasis
A process by which cancer cells migrate and invade surrounding or distant tissues or organs thus spreading the cancer. It is a sign of advanced cancer and generally indicates a poor prognosis.

Metencephalon
Part of the brain comprising the cerebellum and the pons; it is involved in motor control, vestibular control of eye movements, and urinary bladder and respiratory control.

Methemoglobin
An abnormal form of hemoglobin; it has iron in the oxidized, ferric state (Fe^{3+}) in contrast to the normal ferrous (Fe^{2+}) state. Decreased oxygen delivery to the tissues occurs from inability to bind oxygen and by a shift of the oxyhemoglobin dissociation curve to the left. Can be congenital (deficiency of reducing enzymes —methemoglobin reductase) or acquired. Acquired causes are usually drugs such as nitrates (nitroglycerin and nitric oxide, nitrofurantoin) and certain local anesthetics (prilocaine and benzocaine). Severe cases are treated with methylene blue, which reduces methemoglobin back to normal hemoglobin. *Also see oxyhemoglobin dissociation curve (OHDC).*

Methionine
An essential amino acid. Methionine synthase is involved in folate and DNA synthesis and is inhibited by nitrous

oxide (N_2O). May explain the teratogenic effects of N_2O in experimental animals.

Metyrapone

A drug that blocks the conversion of 11-deoxycortisol to cortisol; used in determining the etiology of Cushing's syndrome (pituitary-dependent, adrenal tumors, or ectopic ACTH syndromes). Has been used in the treatment of non-pituitary Cushing's syndrome.

Micelle

A cluster of amphipathic particles formed by the aggregation of molecules; micelles occur in different shapes (spherical, discoidal and cylindrical).

Microglia

See glial cells.

Microvilli

Cytoplasmic finger-like projections from epithelial cells; they contain actin filaments and are found on the apical (luminal) surface of the cells of the small intestine and renal tubules.

Micturition

The process of urination. It is controlled by the micturition reflex which involves sacral parasympathetic nerves. The reflex is initiated by filling of the urinary bladder. Parasympathetic stimulation results in contraction of the detrusor muscle and relaxation of the internal urethral sphincter. Voluntary control of micturition is elicited through contraction of the external urethral sphincter. *Also see urethra.*

Midbrain

The most superior region of the brain stem where reflex centers for visual, auditory and tactile responses are located.

Migraine

An intense paroxysmal unilateral headache associated with systemic symptoms, usually of a visual or gastrointestinal nature. Requires very stringent criteria for diagnosis.

Mineralocorticoids

Hormones secreted by the adrenal cortex; they regulate salt and water balance, which in turn influence blood volume and blood pressure.

Miniature End Plate Potentials (MEPP)

Small spontaneous depolarizations of the post-junctional muscle membrane; occurs even without stimulation of the motor neuron. MEPPs are due to spontaneous discharge of single vesicles (acetylcholine quanta) into the synaptic cleft and are usually too weak to produce a contraction. *Also see Motor end plate potential.*

Minute Ventilation	*See Total Minute Ventilation.*
Mitosis	A type of cell division in which daughter cells receive the exact number of chromosomes and genetic makeup as the parent cell; characteristic of growth and repair processes. *Also see meiosis and telophase.*
Mitral regurgitation	A valvular heart disease in which the mitral valve becomes leaky, allowing blood to return to the left atrium during ventricular systole. Left atrial enlargement results in pulmonary edema and atrial fibrillation in severe cases. Rheumatic heart disease is the most common cause. May also occur after myocardial infarction.
Mitral valve	Miter-shaped heart valve between the left atrium and left ventricle.
Monoamine Oxidase (MAO)	An enzyme present in presynaptic nerve endings; degrades catecholamines and serotonin. MAO inhibition thus enhances transmission at these synapses. MAO inhibitors are used in the treatment of depression (phenelzine and tranylcypromine) and early Parkinson's disease (selegiline). Ingestion of cheese and red wine (rich in tyramine) may result in a hyperadrenergic crisis in patients taking MAOIs. This so called "cheese phenomenon" is due to an inability to metabolize dietary tyramine and other monoamines.
Monoamines	Neurotransmitter molecules having one amino group; e.g. serotonin, dopamine, and norepinephrine.
Monoclonal Antibodies	Identical antibodies produced by a clone of plasma cells; each cell produces identical antibody molecules. They are important in basic science research and medicine and have potential for targeted antimicrobial and cancer treatment. When used as medications, they end in *–mab*.
Monocytes	Largest of the white blood cells; they are non-granular, mononuclear, and phagocytic. In tissues, they differentiate into larger macrophages.
Monoiodotyrosine	Iodized form of tyrosine.
Monokines	Regulatory proteins released by macrophages; they modulate intermediate metabolism, temperature regulation, hormone secretion and immune response.

Mononuclear Leukocyte   Category of leukocytes that includes the lymphocytes and monocytes.

Monosaccharide   A simple sugar; end product of carbohydrate digestion.

Motilin   A neuroactive peptide found in gut and brain tissues.

Motor Cortex   Area of the cortex that influences motor activity; it is made up of three components: Primary motor area, pre-motor area and the supplementary motor area. Axons from the motor cortex constitute the descending pyramidal motor tracts.

Motor Endplate Potential   Excitatory potential produced by massive release of acetylcholine at the post-synaptic membrane of the muscle fiber. It produces muscle contraction. *Also see miniature end plate potential.*

Motor Neuron   A neuron that conducts impulses away from the central nervous system to effector organs (muscles or glands). The interface between a motor neuron and muscle fiber constitutes a specialized type of synapse called the neuromuscular junction.

Motor Neuron Disorders (MND)   A spectrum of neurologic disorders that affects motor neurons. Usually presenting in middle age and seen more commonly in males, it is associated with the progressive destruction of upper and lower motor nerve fibers in the brain and spinal cord, resulting in progressive muscle weakness. Upper motor neuron disease is characterized by spasms and exaggerated reflexes whereas lower motor neuron disease is characterized by progressive wasting (atrophy) and muscle weakness. Amyotrophic lateral sclerosis (ALS), also called Lou Gehrig disease or Charcot's syndrome, is the most common MND. No specific diagnostic test exists and treatment is usually supportive. *Also see upper motor neuron, lower motor neuron, and corticospinal tract.*

Motor Unit   A somatic motor neuron and the group of skeletal muscle fibers that it innervates; an increase in the number of motor units (more muscle fibers per neuron) results in more force generated when activated.

Mucous Membrane   Epithelial lining of the cavities of the digestive, urinary, respiratory and reproductive systems; contains goblet cells which secrete mucus.

Mucous Neck Cells Mucus-secreting cells located in gastric glands.

Müllerian Ducts Also called paramesonephric ducts; they give rise to the accessory reproductive organs in females (uterine canal and Fallopian tubes). They disappear in males.

Müllerian Inhibiting Factor A polypeptide secreted in males by Sertoli cells of the seminiferous tubules; causes regression of the Müllerian ducts.

Multiple Sclerosis A slowly progressive disease of the central nervous system in which there is a breakdown of the protective myelin sheath (demyelination) resulting in progressive neuromuscular deterioration. The exact etiology is unknown but an autoimmune mechanism is suspected.

Murmur See heart murmurs.

Muscarinic Receptor Subtype of acetylcholine receptors. *Also see Acetylcholine.*

Muscle Fiber Muscle unit containing the myofibrils. Skeletal muscle fibers are of two types – based on their speed of contraction: type I fibers (these are slow-twitch fibers) and type II fibers (fast-twitch fibers).

Muscle Spindle A spindle-shaped sensory organ within skeletal muscle that is composed of intrafusal fibers. It is sensitive to muscle stretch and functions as a detector of muscle length.

Muscle Twitch A single contraction of a skeletal muscle – usually observed in the laboratory; it lasts only a fraction of a second and is made up of three components: the latent period, contraction phase and relaxation phase.

Myasthenia Gravis (MG) An autoimmune disease characterized by episodic muscle weakness due to an impairment of neuromuscular transmission. Antibodies are formed against post-junctional acetylcholine receptors resulting in inactivation or destruction. It is most commonly seen in young women and is the best understood autoimmune disease. Babies born to myasthenic mothers may also suffer myasthenia gravis for a brief period and congenital forms have also been described. *Also see acetylcholinesterase and neostigmine.*

Mydriasis Pupillary dilatation resulting from activation of the sympathetic innervation of the eye.

Myelin Sheath

A protective sheath surrounding axons formed by neuroglial cells called *Schwann cells (neurolemmocytes)* in the peripheral nervous system and from oligodendrocytes in the central nervous system. Allows for more rapid transmission of nerve impulses by saltatory conduction. *Also see nodes of Ranvier and saltatory conduction.*

Myeloblasts

Precursor (stem) cells that produce white blood cells.

Myeloma

Malignant tumor of the bone marrow.

Myenteric Plexus

Intrinsic neuronal network located between the longitudinal and circular smooth muscle layers of the walls of the gastrointestinal tract.

Myocardial Infarction

Irreversible necrosis of the heart muscle due to ischemia. Most commonly due to blockage of a major branch of one or both coronary arteries. An important cause of cardiovascular morbidity and mortality.

Myofibrils

Cylindrical organelles located within muscle cells; consist of myofilaments. The myofilaments are of two types: thin filaments (consist of actin) and thick filaments (consist of myosin).

Myogenic regulation

Regulation that maintains a constant blood flow despite varying perfusion pressures (autoregulation). It occurs via changes in vascular smooth muscle tone. This explains the myogenic theory of autoregulation. *Also see autoregulation.*

Myoglobin

A pigmented molecule made up of a single polypeptide chain of 153 amino acid residues; it is found in striated muscles where it serves to store oxygen by binding it to an iron atom. Skeletal muscle damage from any cause can result in the presence of myoglobin in the urine (myoglobinuria), and renal tubular blockage and renal failure may ensue unless adequate hydration is maintained.

Myograph

A device used for the recording of muscle contraction.

Myometrium

The smooth muscle, middle layer of the uterus.

Myoneural Junction

Also called *neuromuscular junction*; the synapse between a motor neuron and the muscle cell that it innervates.

Myopia

Also called *nearsightedness*; it occurs when the eyeball is abnormally long and rays from a distant object are brought into focus in front of the retina. Correction is by use of a biconcave lens. *Also see hyperopia and astigmatism.*

Myoplasm

The intracellular space in muscle cells that contains the contractile elements.

Myosin

The contractile protein that forms the thick filaments; myosin molecule consists of six polypeptide chains: two heavy chains and four light chains. *Also see actin, thick, thin, and intermediate filaments and A-band.*

Myotatic Reflex

Also called *stretch reflex;* a monosynaptic reflex. The stretch reflex has two forms: the *phasic stretch reflex* - elicited by primary afferents of the muscle spindles and *tonic stretch reflex* - elicited by both primary and secondary afferents. The *knee-jerk reflex* is a typical example.

Myotome

Part of the mammalian embryo that forms muscle tissue.

Myxedema

A condition associated with deficiency of thyroid hormone. It is characterized by accumulation of mucoproteins in tissue fluid.

N

Naloxone

A drug that acts as a pure antagonist (no agonist effect) at opioid receptor sites. Used clinically for reversal of opioid-induced respiratory depression by such drugs as morphine and fentanyl. Also reverses analgesia produced by these agents and so must be titrated slowly. Rapid administration of a large dose can result in sympathetic stimulation and this effect has been tried in the treatment of certain types of shock. *Also see opiates.*

Natriuretic Hormone (Atrial)

Also called atrial natriuretic peptide (ANP). *Also see atrial natriuretic factor.*

Natural Killer Cells

Large granular lymphocytes that kill tumor cells and virus-infected cells by cell-to cell contact.

Natural Selection

A Darwinian theory describing the process by which individual members of a population adapt to their specific environment. The theory states that those members who are better able to adapt are more likely to survive and to reproduce.

Nearsightedness

See myopia.

Neck Reflex (Tonic)

A type of positional reflex that is activated by the muscle spindles found in the neck muscles.

Necrosis

Cell death resulting in tissue and organ death; usually due to pathological conditions.

Negative Feedback

A self-regulatory mechanism that serves to maintain a constant internal environment. An example is the process of erythropoiesis: tissue hypoxia stimulates erythropoietin release from the kidneys; erythropoietin stimulates the bone marrow to increase the release of erythropoietin-sensitive stem cells, resulting in an increase in the number of circulating erythrocytes after 2-3 days. This in turn inhibits further release of erythropoietin by the kidneys.

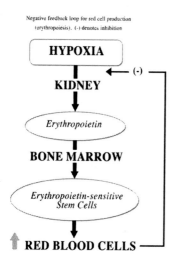

Negative feedback loop for red cell production (erythropoiesis). (-) denotes inhibition

Neoplasm

A new, abnormal growth of tissue as in a tumor.

Neospinothalamic Tract

One of the pain pathways in the spinal cord and brain stem. The type $A\gamma$ fast pain fibers transmit predominantly mechanical and acute thermal pain.

Neostigmine

A quaternary ammonium compound that inactivates acetylcholinesterase; enhances neuromuscular transmission by increasing the amount of acetylcholine at the neuromuscular junction, thus overcoming the competitive inhibition produced by non-depolarizing muscle relaxants. Widely used in anesthetic practice for this purpose. Administered with an antimuscarinic agent such as atropine or glycopyrrolate to avoid untoward muscarinic effects such as bradycardia, bronchospasm, excessive secretions and abdominal pain. *See acetylcholine, acetylcholinesterase and myasthenia gravis.*

Nephron

The functional unit of the kidney; it consists of the individual renal tubule and its glomerulus.

Nernst Equation

An equation that is used to calculate the equilibrium membrane potential for a particular ion of known intracellular and extracellular concentrations:

$$E = \frac{-2.3\,RT}{zF}\,Log_{10}\,\frac{[\,C_i\,]}{[\,C_o\,]}$$

where, E= Equilibrium Potential (mV) and

$$\frac{2.3\,RT}{zF} = \text{Constant (60 mV at } 37^\circ C)$$

z = charge on the ion

C_i = intracellular ion concentration (mM/L)

C_o = extracellular ion concentration (mM/L)

Also see equilibrium potential.

Nerve

A bundle of long fibers and connective tissues of axons in the peripheral nervous system.

Nerve Growth Factor (NGF)

A neurotrophin (stimulant of neuron growth) of particular importance in embryonic development of sensory neurons and sympathetic ganglia. In adult humans, NGF promotes regeneration of neurons after injury. *Also see neurotrophins.*

Nerve Impulse

A propagating nerve action potential.

Neurilemma

The protective Schwann sheath and its surrounding basement membrane; provides a cover for nerve fibers in the peripheral nervous system.

Neuroactive Peptides

See neuropeptides.

Neuroglia

Regarded as supporting cells of the central nervous system. Neuroglial cells ensheath neurons and increase the speed of propagation of action potentials.

Neuroglial Cells

See glial cells.

Neurohormone

A hormone that is released into the blood stream from the nervous system. Examples include: vasopressin, epinephrine, oxytocin and several releasing hormones.

Neurohypophysis

Also called the posterior pituitary gland. It consists mainly of glia-like cells and it stores and secretes antidiuretic hormone and oxytocin produced by the hypothalamus.

Neuromuscular Junction

The synapse between a motor neuron and the sarcolemma of a muscle fiber. Also called the motor end plate. *Also see acetylcholine, acetylcholinesterase and myasthenia gravis.*

Neuron

A highly specialized cell composed of three parts: dendrites, cell body and axon.

Neuropeptide

A class of polypeptides that function as neurotransmitters and neuromodulators. Examples include: Neuropeptide Y, substance P, somatostatin and vasoactive intestinal peptide (VIP).

Neurophysins

Hormones secreted in the hypothalamus from precursors of vasopressin and oxytocin; they function as carrier proteins for vasopressin and oxytocin.

Neurotensin

A brain and gastrointestinal tract neuropeptide present in the brain and enteric neurons. It functions in temperature regulation; induces hypothermia when injected into the cerebrospinal fluid.

Neurotransmitter

A chemical substance synthesized in nerve terminals and stored in synaptic vesicles from where it is released into the synaptic cleft; it acts on the post-synaptic membrane and produces either excitatory or inhibitory postsynaptic potentials.

Neurotrophins

Chemicals that promote neuron growth particularly in the developing fetal brain. In the adult nervous system, neurotrophins are required for regeneration of mature sensory neurons after injury. Examples include: nerve growth factor (NGF) and brain-derived neurotrophic factor. *Also see Nerve growth Factor (NGF).*

Neutropenia

See leukopenia.

Neutrophil

The predominant type of white blood cells; it constitutes the body's first line of defense against infection.

Nexus

A type of cell-to-cell contact as in single-unit smooth muscles.

Niacin

A water-soluble B vitamin required for the formation of the coenzyme, Nicotinamide Adenine Dinucleotide (NAD). Also called nicotinic acid. Deficiency results in a condition called *pellagra*. High dose niacin is used for treating *hypercholesterolemia*.

Nicotinic Receptor

See Acetylcholine.

Nidation

The process of implantation of the blastocyst in the uterine endometrium.

Nifedipine

A dihydropyridine Ca^{2+} channel blocking agent; a widely used antihypertensive agent. *Also see calcium channel blocker.*

Night Blindness

A condition which results from Vitamin A (retinol) deficiency; there is impaired/decreased formation of retinal and consequently, decreased amounts of the photochemical rhodopsin.

Nissl Bodies

Dense-staining areas of rough endoplasmic reticulum contained in the cell body of neurons; it is part of the neuronal biosynthetic apparatus.

Nitric Oxide (NO)

A very potent vasodilator as well as a neurotransmitter in both the central nervous system and in peripheral autonomic neurons. Its biosynthesis occurs in vascular endothelial cells from the precursor L-arginine and by the enzyme NO synthase (NOS). Three isoforms of NOS have been identified. NO has a half-life of a few seconds. Its cellular action is by activation of guanylyl cyclase, which converts guanosine triphosphate (GTP) → cGMP (cyclic guanosine monophosphate), which produces smooth muscle relaxation. NO is now known to mediate a wide range of physiologic functions e.g. blood pressure regulation, intestinal relaxation, long-term potentiation in the brain and penile erection. Neurons that release NO are termed "nitregic" or "nitroxidergic." NO is used in the treatment of persistent pulmonary hypertension of the newborn (PPHN), post cardiopulmonary bypass pulmonary hypertension and Acute lung injury (respiratory distress syndrome) because of its selective pulmonary vasodilating effects. Nitroglycerin and sodium nitroprusside produce vasodilatation by releasing NO. Also the current treatment for erectile dysfunction is with phosphodiesterase type 5 (PDE5) inhibitors that prevent the degradation of cGMP thus promoting penile vessel relaxation and increase blood flow. *Also see EDRF.*

Nociceptors

Pain receptors; they detect physical or chemical damage occurring in the tissues.

Nodes of Ranvier

Gaps in the myelin sheath of myelinated axons, located approximately 1 mm apart, through which action potentials are propagated. Allows for rapid conduction of nerve impulses by saltatory conduction. *Also see myelin sheath and saltatory conduction. Louis Ranvier, French pathologist (1825-1922).*

Non-steroidal Anti-inflammatory Drugs (NSAIDS)

A class of drugs (e.g. aspirin, ibuprofen and ketorolac) that block the cyclooxygenase (COX-1) enzyme and decrease the production of prostaglandins. NSAIDS are effective in the management of inflammation, fever and pain but may cause stomach ulcers since prostaglandins are necessary for gastric protection. Increased bleeding risk likely reflects a decreased amount of thromboxane, which is a potent platelet aggregator. NSAIDS may also affect renal function in compromised patients (especially hypovolemia) by inhibiting autoregulatory mechanisms that are prostaglandin dependent. More specific COX-2 inhibitors lack most of these side effects but appear to have an inherent risk of thrombosis. The

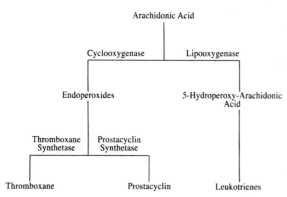

recent association of heart attacks with their chronic use has led to their withdrawal from the market. *Also see cyclooxygenase, thromboxane, and pain.*

Norepinephrine (Noradrenaline)

A catecholamine neurotransmitter with both central and peripheral actions. It is released from postganglionic sympathetic nerve endings. It also acts as a hormone, secreted by the adrenal medulla.

Normoblasts

Intermediate cells in the erythropoietic process; they are mature nucleated cells with condensed nuclear chromatin.

Nuclear Bag Fibers

A type of intrafusal fibers in which the nuclei are arranged in the central region of the fiber. In general, there are two nuclear bag fibers per muscle spindle. *Also see Intrafusal fibers.*

Nuclear Chain Fibers

A type of intrafusal fibers in which the nuclei are arranged in a row along the fiber. In general, there are five to six nuclear chain fibers per muscle spindle. *Also see Intrafusal fibers.*

Nuclear (Hormone) Receptors

Receptors for lipophilic hormones. They function within the nucleus to activate the production of mRNA (genetic transcription). A nuclear hormone receptor is made up of two regions: a ligand (hormone)-binding domain and a DNA-binding domain. Steroids act by binding to specific intracellular receptors at their target site, thus their rather slow onset of action.

Nucleohistone

A nucleoprotein that consists of DNA and a histone.

Nucleolus

Part of the nucleus where ribosomal RNA is produced.

Nucleoplasm

The protoplasm that makes up the nucleus.

Nucleosome

An inactive form of DNA composed of DNA and histone proteins (protein present in chromatin) complex.

Nucleotide

The subunit of the nucleic acids, DNA and RNA; a nucleotide has three subunits: a phosphate group, a five-carbon sugar and a nitrogenous base.

Nucleus

The cellular organelle, centrally-located, and containing the chromosomes; it controls metabolic function and structural characteristics of the cell.

Nutrition

Process by which the body ingests and utilizes nutrients such as: proteins, carbohydrates, fats, minerals, ions, vitamins and water. For daily needs, a balanced diet is necessary. Also, for proper metabolism to occur, energy intake must balance expenditure.

Nystagmus

Rapid oscillatory movements of the eye; usually horizontal but may be vertical. May be due to ocular or extra-ocular diseases.

O

Obesity

Accumulation of excessive amounts of fat in the body. Defined as a Body mass Index (BMI) >29.9kg/m². BMI is the weight in kg divided by the (height in m²).

BMI values are depicted as follows:

20 –24.9 – ideal
25 –29.9 – overweight (pre-obese)
30 – 34.9 – moderate obesity
35 – 39.9 – severe obesity
40 – 49.9 – morbid obesity
>50   super obesity

Obesity results from excessive caloric intake or by other conditions that may be: genetic, hormonal, social or metabolic in origin. Because obesity is associated with various systemic diseases, it is associated with increased morbidity and mortality.

Obstructive Sleep Apnea (OSA)

Cessation of airflow in the upper airways despite respiratory efforts and associated with hemoglobin desaturation. Usually associated with loud snoring and a disturbed sleep pattern and day time somnolence. Results from upper airway obstruction associated with obesity, adenotonsillar hypertrophy and upper airway anomalies. Prolonged OSA can result in significant cardiovascular changes such as systemic and pulmonary hypertension. Diagnosis is by a history, physical examination, and a sleep study (polysomnography). Management strategies include weight loss, use of non-invasive airway devices, and surgery. *Also see apnea.*

Occipital Lobe

The primary area of the cerebral cortex responsible for vision and for the coordination of eye movements.

Odontoblasts

The layer of cells lining the outer wall of the pulp cavity. They are of neural crest origin and function to secrete dentin.

Olestra

An artificial free-fat that tastes, looks and acts like real fat and is not absorbed in the gastrointestinal tract. It is employed in the production of foods free of calories from fat – hence it is sometimes called "fake-fat."

Olfaction

The sense of smell.

Oligodendrocyte

A type of glial cell (supporting cell of the nervous system) that is responsible for the myelination of axons of the central nervous system. *Also see glial cells.*

Oligosaccharides

Short, branched chains of glucose molecules.

Omeprazole

A substituted benzimidazole that irreversibly inhibits the H^+-K^+-ATPase enzyme (proton-pump). This prevents "pumping" of hydrogen ions from the parietal cells and so decreases hydrochloric acid production. Used for the treatment of peptic ulcers, gastro-esophageal reflux disease (GERD) and excessive stomach acid as in Zollinger-Ellison syndrome. *Also see gastritis and peptic ulcer.*

Oncogenes

Genes that promote cancer formation.

Oncology

The medical specialty that deals with the study of cancers and their treatment.

Oncotic Pressure

See colloid osmotic pressure.

Oocyte

An immature egg; there are two types: primary oocyte (which is yet to complete the first meiotic division) and a secondary oocyte (which has commenced the second meiotic division).

Oogenesis

The formation of ova in the ovaries.

Opiates

Derivatives of opium that produce profound analgesia by binding to opiate receptors. Opium is derived from the capsule of the unripe poppy seed-*Papaver somniferum.* Morphine is the prototype opiate against which all other opiates are compared. They are stereo-specifically inhibited by opiate-like compounds that bind to opiate receptors but produce no agonist effects. *Also see naloxone.*

Opportunistic Infection

An infection that occurs because the body's immune system has been severely weakened; opportunistic infections such as pneumonia, tuberculosis and fungal infections pose a major problem in immuno-compromised patients such as HIV/AIDS patients and account for significant morbidity and mortality in these patients.

Opsonization

A term that describes the ability of antibodies to stimulate the process of phagocytosis.

Optic Chiasma

Part of the visual pathway where fibers from the nasal halves of the retina cross over (decussate) to the opposite side and join fibers from the opposite temporal retinas to form the optic tracts. The left visual field is therefore represented on the right side of the brain and vice versa.

Optic Disc

Area of the retina called the blind spot where neurons exit the retina as the optic nerve; it lacks photoreceptors and is also an area for entry and exit of blood vessels.

Optokinetic Reflex

A reflex that allows the eyes to remain fixated on a visual target during head movements.

Oral Contraception

Minimizing the chances of pregnancy through taking birth-control pills; usually, a combination of estrogen and progesterone for 21 days of a 28-day cycle.

Organ

A component of the body comprising two or more primary tissues and is adapted for the performance of a specific function or functions.

Organ of Corti

Also called spiral organ, it is the functional unit of hearing. It is located within the cochlea and consists of hair cells with sensory fibers, the tectoral membrane, and the basilar membrane. It plays a role in the conversion of sound waves into nerve impulses. *Also see cochlea.*

Organelles

Structures within the cytoplasm of cells that perform specialized functions; e.g. Golgi apparatus, endoplasmic reticulum, mitochondria, lysosomes and nucleus.

Orgasm

Associated with the sexual act; in males this occurs during the period of emission and ejaculation and is followed by a refractory period during which another orgasm is physiologically impossible. An increased level of oxytocin is believed to be responsible. In females, orgasm also involves spinal cord reflexes: contractions of the musculature of the perineum, vagina, uterus tubes and also the rectal sphincters. In general, females, unlike males, lack a refractory period.

Orthostatic Hypotension

Also called postural hypotension; usually associated with reduced baroreceptor sensitivity. It is manifested by extreme dizziness or fainting (reduced brain perfusion) on sitting or standing up from the supine position. Clinically it is most commonly used to assess the degree of dehydration or hypovolemia. *A supine hypotensive syndrome* is sometimes seen in advanced pregnancy due to inferior vena cava (IVC) compression by the gravid uterus. Tilting to the left side relieves the symptoms.

Osmoreceptors

Cells located in the hypothalamus and responsible for detection of changes in the osmolality of body fluid.

Osmosis

The movement of water across a semi-permeable membrane from a region of low solute concentration to one of high solute concentration.

Osmotic Pressure

The force required to prevent osmotic movement of water; the greater the solute concentration of a solution the greater the osmotic pressure (the osmotic pressure of water is zero).

Ossicles

Collective name for the three bones in the middle ear (malleus, incus and stapes).

Osteoarthritis

A form of degenerative joint disease (DJD) involving disintegration of the cartilage on the articular surfaces.

Osteoblasts

Bone-forming cells derived from osteoprogenitor cells; they secrete the bone matrix.

Osteocalcin

A 6,000 Dalton molecular mass plasma protein characterized by the presence of γ-carboxyglutamate residues and having a high affinity for calcium. Plasma levels are used as a biomarker of osteoblastic activity.

Osteoclasts

Produced from monocytes; are important for growth and repair of bone.

Osteocytes

Mature bone cells produced from osteoblasts.

Osteomalacia

A bone disorder, particularly in adults, characterized by bone softening from defective mineralization; caused by vitamin D deficiency and other factors.

Osteonectin

A 32,000 Dalton molecular mass protein that binds collagen to form a complex that, in turn binds hydroxyapatite crystals necessary for the bone mineralization process. Over expression of osteonectin has been associated with certain cancers.

Osteoporosis

A bone disorder that occurs most commonly in post-menopausal women; the bones are weakened due to a reduction in bone mass. It may be prevented or its progression slowed by increased dietary intake of vitamin

D and calcium. Secondary types occur in less than 5% of cases.

Osteoprogenitor Cells

Bone stem cells lining the surface of bone: they produce osteoblasts.

Otolith Organs

A part of the vestibular apparatus of the inner ear; made up of the utricle and saccule. *Also see vestibular system.*

Ovarian Follicles

Small structures located in the ovary; contain the ovum and granulosa cells, which secrete estrogen.

Ovary

The reproductive structure in females, responsible for production of ova and the female sex steroids.

Oviduct

Also called the *uterine or fallopian tube;* it is responsible for the transport of ova from the ovaries to the uterus.

Ovulation

The release of mature eggs from the ovarian follicles.

Ovum

The egg cell; located in ovarian follicles. The nucleus combines with a sperm nucleus in the process of fertilization.

Oxidative Phosphorylation

The electron-transport mitochondrial system for adenosine triphosphate (ATP) formation.

Oximeter

A device that measures oxygen saturation of blood. A pulse oximeter is a device used to measure oxygen saturation by measuring the relative absorption of light by oxyhemoglobin and deoxyhemoglobin.

Oxygen content - arterial (C_aO_2)

Amount of oxygen carried by 100 mL of arterial blood. *Also see Appendix I*

Oxygen content - mixed venous (C_vO_2)

Amount of oxygen carried by 100 mL of mixed venous blood. *Also see Appendix I.*

Oxygen Consumption (VO_2)

Denotes oxygen usage by the body. It is about 250 mL per minute at rest for an adult (3-4 mL /kg). Newborns and small children have much higher oxygen consumption (6-8 mL/kg). *Also see Appendix I.*

Oxygen Debt

The extra amount of oxygen consumed during recovery from exercise. It represents the extra oxygen needed for metabolism of the tissues activated during the exercise and oxygen required for the metabolism of lactic acid produced during anaerobic respiration.

Oxygen Delivery (DO₂)

The total amount of oxygen available for delivery to the tissues. Also called oxygen flux. Optimizing oxygen delivery and consumption are considered important concepts in the management of certain critically ill patients. *Also see Appendix I.*

Oxygen extraction ratio (OER)

The percentage of the oxygen content that is utilized by the tissues. *Also see Appendix I.*

Oxyhemoglobin

A compound formed by the combination of oxygen with hemoglobin.

Oxyhemoglobin dissociation curve (OHDC)

The sigmoid-shaped curve that describes the relationship between oxygen saturation and the oxygen tension (PO_2). Some factors e.g. pH shift the curve to the right (decreased affinity and increase oxygen release to the tissues). The opposing factors, as well as fetal hemoglobin, methemoglobin and carboxyhemoglobin shift the curve to the left (increased affinity and decreased oxygen release to tissues). *Also see P_{50}, Bohr effect and Haldane effect.*

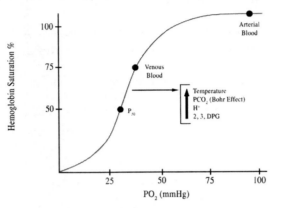

Oxyhemoglobin Dissociation Curve (OHDC)

Oxyhemoglobin Saturation

Usually expressed as a percentage; it denotes the amount of oxyhemoglobin compared to the total amount of hemoglobin in blood. *Also see oximeter.*

Oxyntic Cells

Also called parietal cells; they are present in gastric glands and secrete hydrochloric acid and intrinsic factor. *Also see intrinsic factor and pernicious anemia.*

Oxytocin

A hormone produced in the hypothalamus and stored in the posterior pituitary; it stimulates uterine contractions by a positive feedback mechanism and also stimulates lactation. Synthetic oxytocin is used to augment uterine contractions during labor and after delivery.

Ozone (O₃)

An oxidant present in the atmosphere; inhalation impairs respiration and the nervous system. The ozone layer (located in the lower stratosphere) helps filter out harmful solar ultraviolet radiation.

P

P₅₀

This is the oxygen tension (PO_2) at which hemoglobin is 50% saturated. It is normally 27 mmHg at normal pH and temperature. The P_{50} is a useful indicator of the position of the oxyhemoglobin dissociation curve. A decreased P_{50} indicates a left shift or an increased affinity of hemoglobin for oxygen and vice versa. *Also see oxyhemoglobin dissociation curve.*

p53 (protein 53) gene

A gene that is involved with the regulation of apoptosis (programmed cell death) and slowing or stoppage of the cell cycle when DNA is damaged and requires repair. It is located on the short arm of chromosome 17 in humans. It is, in essence, a tumor suppressor gene and also an important knockout mice model for tumor research. Mutations in this gene are associated with uncontrollable cell division and p53 mutations are present in certain cancer patients. It is a potential target for gene therapy. *Also see gene therapy and knockout mice.*

P Wave

Component of a normal electrocardiogram (EKG). It occurs during atrial systole and signifies atrial depolarization. An absent P wave on the EKG is seen in atrial fibrillation.

Pacemaker

Cardiac cells, characterized by automaticity and rhythmicity; responsible for initiating the heart beat. The sinoatrial (SA) node is the normal pacemaker. Failure of normal pacemaker function or impulse conduction often necessitates an artificial pacemaker.

Pacemaker Potentials

Spontaneous membrane potential changes produced by pacemaker cells of single-unit smooth muscles.

Pacinian corpuscle

Onion-shaped sensory receptor sensitive to pressure and located deep in the dermis.

PAH (Para-Aminohippuric Acid)

A substance used in the assessment of renal function. PAH is filtered and secreted by the nephrons but not reabsorbed. By applying the Fick principle, the clearance of PAH can be calculated and is a measure of the effective renal plasma flow (ERPF).

Pain

The International Association for the Study of Pain (IASP) defines pain as "an unpleasant sensory and emotional experience associated with actual or potential tissue damage or described in terms of such damage." Pain perception is due to response of free nerve endings to noxious stimuli and is transmitted by the A delta and C fibers. Neurotransmitters mediating pain include: glutamate, substance P and Calcitonin gene related protein (CGRP). Bradykinin and prostaglandins are released following tissue damage and further activate free nerve endings, increasing the pain sensation. *Also see non-steroidal anti-inflammatory drugs (NSAIDS) and spinothalamic tract.*

Palpebra

The eyelid.

Palsy (Cerebral)

See cerebral palsy.

Pancreastatin

A 49-amino acid peptide released along with insulin from the β-cell granule; it inhibits insulin secretion and is presumed to play a role in auto feedback regulation of insulin secretion.

Pancreatic Juice

Digestive juice secreted by the pancreas; it contains bicarbonate ions and the enzymes: trypsin, lipase, and amylase.

Papillary Muscles

Muscles holding the atrioventricular valves to the ventricular walls.

Pap test (smear)

A method of staining smears of various body secretions to detect the presence of abnormal cells in exfoliated cells. Most common application is in the detection of early cervical cancer. Named after Greek American physician and anatomist – *George Nicolas Papanicolaou (1883 -1962)*

Paracellular pathway

The leakage of water and other solutes through tight junctions as occurs in renal tubular epithelium, small intestine, and gallbladder.

Paracrine Regulator

Chemical messenger produced within one tissue and regulates a different tissue of the same organ; e.g. the endothelium of blood vessels produces substances that cause the smooth muscles to contract or relax.

Paranasal sinuses

Air-filled chambers with a mucous membrane lining; communicate with the lateral wall of the nasal cavity. There are four pairs: maxillary, sphenoid, frontal and ethmoidal sinuses. They become fully developed in the teenage years.

Paraplegia

Paralysis of the lower half of the body (below the waist) due to spinal cord injury; other causes include poliomyelitis, spinal tuberculosis, syphilis and spinal tumors.

Parasympathetic Nervous System (PNS)

Also called the "cranio-sacral" division of the autonomic nervous system: long preganglionic fibers originate in the cranial parts- cranial nerves III (oculomotor), VII (facial), IX (glossopharyngeal) and X (vagus) and the sacral part of the spinal cord. These terminate on ganglia close to or within the effector organs. Short postganglionic fibers innervate visceral organs. The vagus nerve provides parasympathetic innervation to the heart, esophagus, stomach, small intestine, liver, upper half of the large intestine and lungs. Sacral Parasympathetic fibers innervate terminal ganglia in the lower half of the large intestine, the rectum, and the genitourinary systems. *Also see autonomic nervous system and sympathetic nervous system.*

Parathyroid Hormone (PTH)

A polypeptide hormone secreted by the parathyroid glands. It regulates calcium and phosphate metabolism. Plasma Ca^{2+} is raised by:

- Increased bone resorption and increased osteoclastic activity.
- Increased Ca^{2+} reabsorption by the distal tubules of the kidney
- Increased formation of 1,25-dihydroxycholecalciferol, which increases Ca^{2+} absorption from the intestine.

PTH decreases plasma phosphate levels by increasing urinary phosphate excretion. *Also see Calcitonin and resorption.*

Parietal Cell

See oxyntic cells.

Parietal Lobe

Portion of the cerebral cortex (somatic sensory cortex) that lies immediately behind the central fissure; it has two subdivisions, separated by the intra-parietal sulcus: superior parietal lobule and the inferior parietal lobule. The parietal lobe is involved in the integration of sensory information from various senses and in the manipulation of objects as well as visuo-spatial processing.

Parkinson's disease

A condition characterized by tremors of resting muscles; it is caused by inadequate dopamine-producing neurons in the basal ganglia. Also called paralysis agitans. *Also see basal ganglia.*

Parotid glands

A pair of large salivary glands located below and in front of the ears; secretes salivary juice containing water, salts and salivary amylase.

Paroxysmal Tachycardia

Sudden, rapid, rhythmic discharge of impulses spreading in all directions throughout the heart; it is most commonly caused by "re-entry" mechanisms. Conduction through an accessory pathway such as the bundle of Kent is another cause of paroxysmal tachycardia. When hemodynamic instability occurs, direct current (DC) cardioversion is required to immediately restore sinus rhythm and slow the heart rate.

Parturition

The process comprising labor and childbirth.

Passive Immunity

See immunization.

Passive transport

The movement of substances from an area of higher concentration to one of lower concentration. It is independent of energy expenditure.

Pasteur Effect

Describes the decreased glucose utilization and lactic acid production in tissues or organisms when exposed to oxygen.

Patent Ductus Arteriosus

See ductus arteriosus.

Pathogen

Any disease-producing agent.

Pedicle

The part of a vertebra that attaches the posterior aspect of the vertebral body to the lamina. There are two pedicles per vertebra.

Pentagastrin

A synthetic gastrin composed of the terminal four amino acids of gastrin plus alanine: Can perform the actions of gastrin, cholecystokinin and secretin. It is used as a testing agent for the diagnosis of diseases of the stomach. *Also see gastrin.*

Pepsin

The protein-splitting enzyme secreted in gastric juice by gastric glands.

Peptic ulcer

An injury to the mucosal linings of the esophagus, stomach or small intestine; caused by the action of hydrochloric acid (HCL) and pepsin in gastric juice.

Chronic gastritis associated with Helicobacter pylori infection is often associated with peptic ulcers. Another important cause is the chronic use of non-steroidal anti-inflammatory drugs (NSAIDS) such as aspirin and related drugs. *Also see pyrosis, gastritis, and omeprazole.*

Peptidases

Gastrointestinal enzymes that split small peptides into amino acids.

Perfusion

Denotes the flow of blood through an organ. Perfusion pressure in any organ is the mean arterial pressure (MAP) minus the mean venous pressure. This is an important concept in understanding regional blood flow to various organs especially the vital organs (heart, brain, and kidneys).

Pericardium

A serous membrane that surrounds and protects the heart. Collection of significant amounts of fluid can cause pericardial tamponade, a very serious medical emergency.

Perichondrium

A layer of toughened connective tissue sheet that covers cartilaginous structures.

Perikaryon

The neuronal cell body.

Perilymph

The fluid present in the space between the membranous and osseous (bony) labyrinths of the inner ear; it provides a medium for the vibrations involved in hearing and the maintenance of equilibrium.

Perimetrium

The outer serosal layer of the uterine wall.

Perimysium

The connective tissue sheath surrounding bundles of skeletal muscle fibers.

Periosteum

Fibrous connective tissue that covers the surface of bones; it contains blood and lymphatic vessels, nerves and osteoblasts, needed for new bone formation.

Peripheral Chemoreceptors

Chemoreceptors located in the carotid and aortic bodies; they are sensitive to decreased pO_2, increased pCO_2, and decreased pH. In contrast, central chemoreceptors are located in the medulla and are mostly sensitive to CO_2 and pH changes.

Peripheral Nervous System (PNS)

The portion of the nervous system comprising the cranial nerves (from the brain) and spinal nerves (from the spinal cord). *Also see central nervous system.*

Peripheral Resistance

Denotes the resistance to blood flow through the arterial system; the resistance to blood flow is inversely proportional to the fourth power of the radius (r^4) of the vessel. *Also see Total peripheral resistance and Hagen-Poiseuille's law.*

Peristalsis

Rhythmic contractions of smooth muscles of tubular organs, e.g. the digestive tract. It serves to propel the contents towards the ano-rectum.

Peritonitis

Inflammation of the peritoneum. Common causes are perforated viscus, localized infections of intra-abdominal organs, acute hemorrhage into the peritoneum and certain chronic diseases like liver cirrhosis or tuberculosis. Initially, visceral peritonitis produces poorly localized abdominal pain referred to the umbilicus. As the infection continues, parietal peritonitis produces more severe pain, which is localized to the affected area. Ultimately, this will progress to diffuse peritonitis with involuntary guarding of abdominal muscles causing a "rigid" abdomen. *Also see visceral peritoneum.*

Peritubular Capillaries

A capillary bed that surrounds the nephron; the peritubular capillaries run into the peritubular veins which in turn drain into the interlobular veins, arcuate veins, interlobar veins, renal vein and inferior vena cava. Peritubular capillaries serve to reabsorb nutrients and plasma extracted in the Bowman's capsule.

Permissive Effect

A phenomenon in which a hormone enhances the responsiveness of a target organ to a second hormone or when a hormone potentiates the action of a second hormone. Glucocorticoids exert a permissive effect for the metabolic and other actions of catecholamines.

Pernicious Anemia

Megaloblastic anemia resulting from the lack of intrinsic factor secretion by gastric parietal cells; it is characterized by a lack of absorption of vitamin $B_{12,}$ an essential factor in the formation of red blood cells. *Also see anemia and intrinsic factor.*

Petit Mal (Epilepsy)

A seizure disorder most common in adolescents and children (usually above five years), characterized by 3 to 30 seconds of unconsciousness with twitch-like muscle contractions usually in the head region; it involves the reticular activating system. The EEG shows typical 3/

second spikes. Also called *absence seizures*; the patient is normal between seizures. *Also see epilepsy and grand mal seizures.*

pH

A term that describes the hydrogen ion (H^+) concentration of a solution. Mathematically, it is the negative logarithm of the hydrogen ion concentration. The pH scale in common use ranges from 0 to 14. Solutions with a pH of 7 are neutral; those with a pH lower than 7 are acidic; and those higher than 7 are basic. Normal blood pH ranges from 7.35 to 7.45. A normal pH of 7.40 corresponds to a hydrogen ion concentration of 40 nmol/liter. Precise pH regulation is necessary for chemical reactions and enzymatic activity to proceed unimpeded. *Also see Henderson-Hasselbalch equation, buffer, acidosis and alkalosis.*

Phagocytosis

The process of engulfing bacteria and/or debris; cellular ingestion.

Pharyngoesophageal sphincter

See upper esophageal sphincter.

Pharynx

Part of the gastrointestinal and respiratory tracts located between the mouth and the esophagus; it consists of three parts: nasopharynx, oropharynx, and laryngopharynx (hypopharynx). The pharynx also plays an important role in phonation.

Phenotype

An individual's physical or observable traits; e.g. brown or blue eyes. The genotype, on the hand, is the genetic makeup of the individual or cell.

Phenylalanine

An essential amino acid and the precursor for L-dopa, dopamine, norepinephrine, and epinephrine.

Phenylketonuria (PKU)

An autosomal recessive genetic disorder of metabolism that results from a defect in the enzyme that converts the amino acid phenylalanine to tyrosine (phenylalanine hydroxylase). It is associated with mental delay and if detected early, can be prevented with artificial diet low in phenylalanine. A screening test is performed on most newborns in developed countries.

Pheromone

A substance secreted to the outside of the body by most mammals; they help in the regulation of their reproductive cycles and behavior and also alter the behavior of animals of the same species.

Phonocardiography

A record of the acoustics or heart sounds during the cardiac cycle.

Phonocardiogram

A graphic record of the heart sounds and murmurs produced by blood flow. Obtained by applying a microphone on the chest; it has now been surpassed by more modern techniques like echocardiography and is now largely of historical interest.

Phorbol Esters

Highly irritant and tumor-promoting compounds obtained from plants; they activate protein kinase C enzyme.

Phosphodiesterase

The enzyme that catalyzes the breakdown of phosphodiester bonds present in nucleic acids. It splits cyclic AMP into inactive products, thus inhibiting the second messenger function of cyclic AMP. There are 5 subtypes of phosphodiesterase enzyme (PDE1, PDE2, PDE3, PDE4 and PDE5). Phosphodiesterase inhibitors (PDIs) potentiate the action of cyclic AMP and are used in clinical practice as inotropes (amrinone, milrinone) and as bronchodilators (aminophyline, theophylline). Caffeine and aminophylline are non-selective PDE inhibitors. *Also see cAMP, adenylyl cyclase and theophylline.*

Phospholipids

A major lipid component of cell membranes; it is composed of fatty acids, glycerol and a phosphate group. In the alveoli, phospholipids function as surfactants. Sphingomyelin and phosphoglycerides are two types of phospholipids with sphingosine and glycerol backbones, respectively.

Phosphorylation

The process whereby an inorganic phosphate group is added to an organic molecule; e.g. the addition of a phosphate group to ADP to generate ATP from creatine phosphate.

Photopic vision

Also called bright light (daylight) vision; it is usually a function of cones, which generally have a much higher threshold and greater acuity.

Photopsin

Protein components of photochemicals found in cones; necessary for photopic or color vision.

Photoreceptors

Light-sensitive sensory receptors (rods and cones) located in the retina.

Physostigmine (Eserine)

A naturally occurring anticholinesterase drug derived from the Calabar bean, the seed of *physostigma venenosum*. It is indigenous to West Africa and was once used by local tribes in "trial by ordeal". Unlike neostigmine and pyridostigmine, it is a tertiary amine and so crosses the blood-brain barrier and placenta. It is used in the treatment of central anticholinergic syndrome and to reverse the sedative effects of benzodiazepines, phenothiazines and tricyclic antidepressants. It also reverses the respiratory depressant effects of opioids. It also produces miosis and is used as eye drops for the treatment of glaucoma. It is no longer used for reversal of neuromuscular blockade because of its generalized actions. Also called *antilirium*. *Also see acetylcholinesterase.*

Pia mater

The highly vascular and delicate innermost of the three layers of the connective tissue (meninges) covering the central nervous system. The outer layers are the arachnoid mater and the dura mater.

Piloerector muscles

The muscles located in the skin which, upon contraction, makes the hairs stand erect; they are innervated by sympathetic cholinergic fibers.

Pinna

The outer cartilaginous structure of the external ear; *also called the auricle.*

Pineal Gland

A gland located in the third ventricle. It secretes melatonin in response to sensory signals from the photoreceptors.

Pinocytosis

A nonspecific process performed by many cells in which the cell membrane invaginates to form a deep furrow which fuses to form a vesicle containing extracellular fluid.

Pituicytes

Small branching glial cells present in the posterior lobe of the pituitary gland; they are presumed to regulate the release of oxytocin and arginine vasopressin.

Pituitary Gland

Also called the *hypophysis;* it is a small endocrine gland about 1 cm in diameter. It is connected to the hypothalamus by a stalk-like structure. The pituitary gland is functionally divided into an anterior pituitary (secretes ACTH, TSH, FSH, LH, growth hormone and prolactin) and a posterior pituitary (secretes oxytocin and antidiuretic hormone).

pK

It is the negative logarithm (to base 10) of the dissociation constant (K_d).

Placenta

The connection between the mother and the developing fetus; necessary for fetal nutrition and circulation. It also has hormonal functions: it secretes human chorionic gonadotropin (HCG), human chorionic somatomammotropin (HCS) progesterone, estrogen, and gonadotropin-releasing hormone (GnRH), all necessary for the growth and survival of the fetus.

Plasma

The liquid component of blood, representing 55% of whole blood or 5% of the body weight. It contains water and inorganic and organic substances. *Serum* is plasma that is devoid of fibrinogen and other clotting factors.

Plasma cells

Cells found in lymphoid tissues and derived from B lymphocytes that are responsible for mass production of antibodies. *Also see humoral immunity and B-cell lymphocytes*

Plasmalemma

The cell membrane. It surrounds the cytoplasm and regulates entry and exit of molecules from the cell.

Plasmin

See fibrinolysin and fibrinolysis.

Platelet

Fragments of giant cells (megakaryoctes) derived from bone marrow. Platelets circulate in the blood and form a plug that seals damaged blood vessels. They play an important role in the hemostatic process. Clopidogrel (Plavix) is an oral antiplatelet agent that is used for clot prevention in patients with coronary artery disease, strokes, and peripheral vascular disease. It acts by inhibiting an ADP chemoreceptor.

Pleural cavity

The potential space between the parietal and visceral pleura. Accumulation of fluid in this space is called a pleural effusion and accumulation of air is called a pneumothorax. *Also see intrapleural space and pneumothorax.*

Pleural Pressure

Pressure of fluid in the space between the chest wall (parietal) pleura and the lung (visceral) pleura. Normal pleural pressure is approximately -5cm H_2O. Excessive positive pleural pressure from accumulation of fluid or air can result in lung collapse.

Pluripotent (stem) cells

Stem cells which can develop into any of the following tissue types: endoderm (interior lining of the gut), mesoderm (blood bone and muscle) and ectoderm (epidermal tissues and nervous system). There are two types of stem cells: embryonic and adult stem cells (blood-forming cells in the bone marrow). Bone marrow transplantation is an established treatment for certain leukemias, cancers and certain metabolic diseases. Stem cell research with a focus on cell-based therapies is a very active area of interest. If ultimately successful, it would be possible to induce stem cells to differentiate into the specific cell type required to repair damaged adult tissue. A possible translation of this research is the potential to treat neurologic injury by making nerve cells from stem cells.

Pneumocytes

Specialized epithelial cells lining the alveolar walls; there are two types: Type I and Type II pneumocytes. Type II pneumocytes produce surfactant and have the ability to differentiate into Type I cells. Type I cells possess special connections with alveolar capillaries, which enhance gaseous diffusion. *Also see Hyaline membrane disease and surfactant.*

Pneumotaxic center

One of the neural respiratory centers, located in the pons and superior to the respiratory center in the medulla. It switches off inspiration by inhibiting neuronal signals in the phrenic nerve. The pneumotaxic center rhythmically antagonizes the apneustic center. A normal rhythm of breathing persists in the absence of this center. *Also see apneustic center.*

Pneumothorax

The presence of free air in the pleural cavity. Common causes include chest trauma, invasive positive pressure ventilation (*barotrauma*) and central venous cannulation. May also occur spontaneously without prior trauma. Also associated with certain underlying pulmonary diseases and certain surgical procedures. When air continues to enter the pleural space and is unable to escape, a *tension pneumothorax* occurs. This results in total lung and cardiovascular collapse unless the pleural space is rapidly decompressed with a needle and/or a chest tube. *Also see pleural cavity and intrapleural space.*

Podocytes

Also called foot cells, they are located in the glomerulus

of the Bowman's capsule; they help in the filtration process and prevent the filtration of proteins.

Poiseuille Equation

See Hagen-Poiseuille Equation.

Polar Bodies

Small daughter cells produced by meiosis; they undergo degeneration during the process of oocyte production and represent a way to discard unnecessary chromosomes while retaining much of the cytoplasm in the ovum.

Polycystic ovary syndrome

A syndrome in which there is LH-dependent hyperandrogenism with irregular menstruation, obesity and development of male type hair distribution. There is a persistent elevation of the LH/FSH ratio. *Also called Stein-Leventhal syndrome.*

Polycythemia

An increased hemoglobin concentration (usually a hematocrit > 64%) and increased red blood cell mass (erythrocytosis). Classified as primary (polycythemia rubra vera) or secondary. Secondary causes include: newborn state, hypoxic states (high altitude, cardiac disease and pulmonary disease), abnormal hemoglobins, and hormone-related causes as in renal disease and certain functional tumors. A decrease in plasma volume, as may occur in acute dehydration, results in *hemoconcentration* and *not* true polycythemia. Correction of dehydration results in normalization of the hematocrit. Polycythemia is associated with increased blood viscosity and an increased risk of thrombosis.

Polydipsia

Excessive thirst associated with an increased fluid intake. A common feature of uncontrolled diabetes mellitus (DM), diabetes insipidus (DI) but may also be of psychogenic origin.

Polymer

Synthetic or naturally-occurring molecule consisting of repeated smaller subunits called monomers.

Polymorphonuclear Leukocyte

A granular leukocyte containing a nucleus and a number of lobes connected by thin cytoplasmic strands. Includes neutrophils, eosinophils, and basophils.

Polyneuritis

Inflammation of several peripheral nerves. It is often associated with paralysis, pain, and muscle wasting.

Polyp

A benign tumor found in the linings of mucous

membranes especially in the nasal cavity, gastrointestinal tract, bladder and uterus.

Polypeptide

A peptide containing a chain of amino acids linked by peptide bonds; one or more polypeptides constitute a protein. Polypeptides are formed during the process of translation.

Polyphagia

Excessive eating.

Polyposis

The presence of multiple polyps. Associated with malignant transformation in certain types and locations e.g. intestinal polyposis.

Polysaccharide

A carbohydrate comprising covalently-bonded monosaccharides; e.g. glycogen and starch.

Polyunsaturated fat

A type of fat found in vegetable oils and margarines that tends to lower blood cholesterol levels.

Polyuria

Excretion of large volumes of urine; commonly associated with uncontrolled diabetes mellitus, diabetes insipidus, chronic renal disease and diuretic use.

Pons

The area between the medulla and brainstem or midbrain; contains the pontine nuclei and the respiratory centers (apneustic and pneumotaxic centers).

Portal System

An array of blood vessels consisting of two capillary beds arranged in series: venous blood from the first capillary bed supplies a second capillary bed before returning to the heart; an example is the hepatic portal system. Portal hypertension is a major complication of liver cirrhosis. *Also see hepatic circulation and cirrhosis.*

Positive Feedback

Homeostatic response mechanism that produces amplification of an initial change; for example, activation of the clotting process activates numerous other clotting factors in a cascade fashion.

Posterior Pituitary Gland

An endocrine gland, which secretes antidiuretic hormone (ADH) and oxytocin. *Also see pituitary gland.*

Postsynaptic Inhibition

The inhibition of synaptic transmission by the action of inhibitory postsynaptic potentials (IPSP). Hyperpolarization of the postsynaptic membrane occurs.

Postural Reflex

Also called the *positive supportive reaction.* The reflex

Potassium Channels

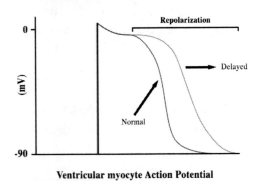

Ventricular myocyte Action Potential

helps position a subject, often in a standing position, prepare for movement/locomotion.

Channels in the cell membrane through which potassium ions enter or leave the cell. They have been classified as fast and slow but other more complex classifications and sub classifications exist based on their function, structure and activation. Potassium-channel blockers (Amiodarone, Sotalol, and Bretylium) are Class III antiarrhythmic compounds which bind to and block potassium channels. By prolonging repolarization, they increase the duration of the action potential and the effective refractory period.

Precordial Leads

Unipolar chest leads used in ECG recording. They comprise six chest leads (V1-V6) recorded with an exploring electrode. They are placed from the right fourth intercostal space to the sixth rib on the left. V1 and V2 record events in the right heart, V3 and V4 record events in the interventricular septum and V5 and V6 record the left side of the heart. *Also see Einthoven's triangle*

Prednisone

A synthetic steroid that possesses glucocorticoid and mineralocorticoid activity.

Preeclampsia

Hypertension, proteinuria and/or edema associated with pregnancy. Also known as *toxemia of pregnancy*, it is a significant cause of maternal morbidity and mortality. *Also see eclampsia.*

Pregnenolone

An important precursor in the formation of adrenocortical hormones; it is converted from cholesterol by cholesterol desmolase under the influence of luteinizing hormone (LH) or adrenocorticotrophic hormone (ACTH).

Prehormone

The inactive form of a hormone; it is converted to the active form within the target cell.

Preload

Refers to the "load" or force applied to a muscle before it contracts. When used in reference to the cardiovascular system, it refers to the stretch or "load" on the ventricles at the end of diastole, just prior to systolic ejection. This is the end diastolic volume (EDV) or pressure. Clinically, this is the pulmonary capillary wedge pressure (PCWP) for the left heart and the central venous pressure (CVP) for the right heart.

Presbyopia

A visual defect caused by the recession of the near point of vision due to increased hardness of the lens. Usually associated with advancing age, there is a progressive loss of accommodation. Correction is by the use of a convex lens.

Presynaptic Inhibition

A form of synaptic inhibition in which axo-axonic synapses inhibit the release of neurotransmitters from the presynaptic axon.

Proaccelerin

A clotting factor also called *Factor V, labile factor or accelerator globulin;* necessary for normal clotting. Deficiency of this factor, usually congenital, results in *parahemophilia.*

Process Cell

Any thin cytoplasmic extension of a cell such as neuronal dendrites and axons.

Prodrug

An inactive form of a drug that must undergo chemical conversion in the body to become active. An example is the ACE inhibitor, *enalapril,* which is hydrolyzed to the active form *enalaprilat.*

Progesterone

A female sex steroid hormone secreted by the corpus luteum and the placenta; it is necessary for preparing the body for pregnancy and maintenance of pregnancy. Progesterone acts on progesterone receptors on target cells e.g. the endometrium. The hormone-receptor complex binds to a progesterone response element in the cell nucleus.

Progestins

Synthetic derivatives of progesterone.

Prohormone

The less-active precursor of a polypeptide hormone that is produced within the cells of an endocrine gland; it undergoes conversion into the active hormone by an enzymatic process prior to secretion of the hormone. An example is parathyroid hormone (PTH).

Prolactin

A hormone secreted by the anterior pituitary gland that stimulates and maintains milk production from the mammary glands. Prolactin secretion displays diurnal variation: the serum concentration rises during sleep and falls while awake. Measurement of prolactin levels is used in the investigation of disorders of the anterior pituitary gland, the hypothalamus, and infertility.

Pronormoblast The stage, during erythropoiesis, preceding the formation of the normoblast; during this stage, the red blood cell still possesses its organelles.

Proprioceptors Sensory receptors that deliver information about body position and movement to the brain; Examples include: Golgi tendon organs, joint receptors, and muscle spindles.

Prorenin The inactive form and precursor of renin; it is stored in the juxtaglomerular cells of the kidney.

Prostaglandins Twenty-one-carbon fatty acids (eicosanoids) formed from phospholipids via arachidonic acid, in response to various stimuli. They possess a variety of functions including stimulation of uterine contractions, gastric acid secretion, and are potent mediators of inflammation. *Also see eicosanoids, cyclooxygenase and non-steroidal anti inflammatory drugs (NSAIDS).*

Protanopia A form of color blindness in which the affected individual is unable to distinguish the color red. It is due to defects in the red cones.

Protein Kinase An enzyme that is involved in signal transduction processes that regulate enzymatic activity. There are two types (A and C) and they possess different isoforms. Protein kinase phosphorylates amino acid residues and is activated by Ca^{2+}-Calmodulin, cAMP, and diacylglycerol (DAG).

Proteins Large organic molecules composed of amino acid subunits that are linked by peptide bonds.

Prothrombin Clotting factor II, the precursor of thrombin. It is produced in the liver. *Also see clotting factors, thrombin, fibrinolysis and fibrinolysin.*

Protoplasm The colloidal semi-fluid complex of a cell consisting of proteins, fats and aqueous suspensions; it also includes the cytoplasm and nucleoplasm.

Pruritus Itching from any cause. May result from a primary skin condition, systemic disease, or may be drug induced.

Pseudohermaphrodite An old terminology used to describe an individual who has the genetic and gonadal composition of one sex but possesses secondary sexual characteristics of the opposite sex. Now referred to as *intersexual* or *ambiguous genitalia. Also see hermaphrodite.*

Pseudopod

A temporary foot-like projection of the cytoplasm common in some cells with ameboid motion; it serves as an organ of locomotion and feeding by the process of phagocytosis.

Pseudoptosis

A reduction in the size of the palpebral aperture.

Ptyalin

An enzyme present in salivary juice that breaks down starch into smaller molecules; also called *salivary amylase. Also see salivary glands.*

Puberty

Denotes attainment of adulthood and is associated with the development of secondary sexual characteristics and reproductive potential.

Pulmonary Circulation

Denotes blood circulation through the lungs; it consists of the right heart, the pulmonary arteries, capillaries and veins. Deoxygenated blood flows into the lungs via the pulmonary arteries while oxygenated blood flows into the left atrium via the pulmonary veins. Ventricular contraction then pumps blood into the systemic circulation. Pressure in the pulmonary circulation is much lower than in the systemic circulation resulting in a lower vascular resistance (PVR). Measurement of the pulmonary capillary wedge pressure (PCWP) using a specialized catheter is used as an indicator of left heart filling pressures and left ventricular function, when certain conditions are met. *Also see systemic circulation and central venous pressure (CVP).*

Pulse Pressure

The difference between the systolic and diastolic blood pressures. It is 40-50mmHg in a normal adult. *Also see mean arterial pressure (MAP).*

Pupil

An opening in the center of the iris that provides a channel for the transmission of light to the retina.

Pupillary Light Reflex

Unilateral pupillary constriction in response to light; constriction of the contralateral pupil is called consensual light reflex. Certain disease conditions such as syphilis may cause a loss of this reflex.

Purkinje Fibers

Specialized cardiac impulse-conducting tissues; *Also see Cardiac Conduction System.*

Pyloric glands   Glands present in the antrum of the stomach. There are two types: G cells, which secrete gastrin and mucous neck cells, which secrete mucus, pepsinogen, and bicarbonate ions.

Pyloric sphincter   A sphincter located at the gastro-duodenal junction.

Pyramidal Tract   *See corticospinal tracts and descending pathways.*

Pyrexia   *See fever and hyperpyrexia.*

Pyrogen   A fever-producing agent. Common examples are bacterial endotoxin and certain inflammatory mediators. *Also see fever.*

Pyrosis   Also called *heartburn*; A burning sensation in the upper abdomen or mid chest caused by acid reflux into the lower esophagus. *Also see gastritis, peptic ulcer, and omeprazole.*

Pyruvic acid   Intermediate product of carbohydrate metabolism.

Q

QRS Complex

The principal deflection of an electrocardiogram; produced by ventricular depolarization. *Also see ECG.*

Q-T interval

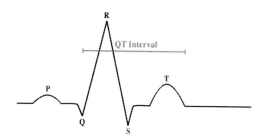

The interval between the beginning of the QRS complex and the end of the T-wave on a standard ECG tracing; it denotes the duration of electrical activity in the ventricles. The Q-Tc is the Q-T interval corrected for heart rate. Long QT syndrome (LQTS) results from prolonged repolarization and is a rare but important cause of life-threatening *tachyarrhythmias*. It may be inherited or acquired (usually medication-induced).

Quadrantanopia

Also called *quadrantic hemianopia*; A condition in which there is visual loss in a quarter of the visual field of one or both eyes.

Quantal release

Secretion of packets of neurotransmitters through the presynaptic membrane at a neuromuscular junction. *Also see acetylcholine.*

R

R wave	A component of the QRS complex of the electrocardiogram. *Also see QRS complex.*
Rapid eye movement (REM) sleep	The rapid movement of the eyes that occurs during the lightest stage of sleep. It is comparable to the awake state. In a typical night sleep, there are 4-5 periods of REM sleep which add up to 90-120 minutes. REM sleep is characterized by active dreams and strong muscular movement.
Ratchet theory (of muscle contraction)	A hypothesis regarding muscle contraction that involves the attachment of cross-bridges from the myosin filaments to the active sites of the activated actin filament. The force of contraction is directly proportional to the degree of interaction between the myosin cross-bridges and the activated actin filament.
Rate receptors	Rapidly-adapting sensory receptors such as joint receptors; they respond to changes in stimulus strength but do not respond to sustained stimuli.
Rathke's pouch	Embryonic invagination of the pharyngeal epithelium from which the anterior pituitary gland originates. Normally closes early in fetal life but persists as a cyst or cleft which may give rise to a suprasellar brain tumor called *craniopharyngioma*. *(Martin Heinrich Rathke, German Anatomist, 1793-1860)*
Reactive hyperemia	The transient rise in blood flow to an organ that follows a short period of blood flow interruption. *Also see functional hyperemia.*
Receptive Field	An area of the peripheral sensory space whose stimulation results in the activation of a particular sensory neuron.
Recessive allele	An allele that expresses its phenotypic effect in the homozygous state but not in the presence of a dominant allele.
Reciprocal Inhibition	A phenomenon associated with muscle stretch: the stretch reflex in a limb elicits reciprocal inhibition of antagonist muscles. The neuronal pathway involves the muscle spindle afferents, which synapse with α-motor neurons that innervate the antagonist muscles.

Recruitment (motor units)

The phenomenon of successive activation of motor units associated with increasing strength of skeletal muscle contraction. Two types are described: spatial recruitment (the number of active motor units is increased) and temporal recruitment (the rate of firing of individual motor units increases). Motor units are normally recruited according to their sizes, starting with the smallest.

Reduced Hemoglobin

See deoxyhemoglobin.

Reflex

An instantaneous involuntary response to a stimulus. *Also see spinal reflex.*

Refraction

The deflection of light rays as they pass between media of different densities.

Refractory Period

The period of time in which an excitable tissue (muscle or nerve) is resistant to activation. Two types are described: *absolute refractory period* – denotes the period immediately following an excitation in which a second stimulus, no matter how great in intensity, cannot elicit a response. The *relative refractory period* denotes the period shortly after an excitation, when there is partial repolarization and a stimulus of normal or greater intensity can elicit a second response. *Also see action potential.*

Releasing Hormones

Polypeptide hormones secreted by the hypothalamus; they stimulate the anterior pituitary gland to release specific hormones.

REM sleep

See rapid eye movement sleep.

Renal Clearance

The volume of plasma that is completely cleared of a particular substance by the kidneys per minute. Renal clearance of a substance provides an estimate of glomerular filtration rate (GFR), provided the substance is neither secreted nor reabsorbed by the renal tubules e.g. inulin. *See glomerular filtration rate and inulin.*

Renal Cortex

The outer granular region of the kidney.

Renal failure

A severe impairment of renal function. Two types exist: (a) Acute renal failure: the kidneys abruptly stop working but normal functioning may resume if treated promptly. (b) Chronic renal failure: involves progressive loss of function of increasing numbers of nephrons and eventually progressing to end-stage renal disease (ESRD). Also classified as pre-renal (hypovolemia), renal and post-renal (obstructive).

Renal medulla

The inner part of the kidney. It contains the renal pyramids.

Renal pelvis

Cavity in the renal medulla through which urine flows to the ureters.

Renal Pyramids

Pyramidal structures visible in longitudinal sections of the kidney; they contain part of the secreting tubules and collecting tubules of the renal medulla.

Renal tubule

Part of the nephron which extends from the renal corpuscle to the collecting duct.

Renin

A proteolytic enzyme secreted by the juxtaglomerular apparatus of the kidneys; it activates the renin-angiotensin system catalyzing the conversion of angiotensinogen to angiotensin I. Also called angiotensinogenase. *Also see angiotensin II, Angiotensin Converting Enzyme (ACE), and juxtaglomerular apparatus.*

Rennin

A proteolytic enzyme that coagulates milk; it is synthesized by chief cells in gastric glands in infants. Also called chymosin.

Replication

The process by which exact copies of a DNA molecule are produced.

Repolarization

The process by which the resting membrane potential of an excitable tissue is re-established after the depolarization phase of an action potential. It is due to an increased permeability of the membrane to potassium ions. *Also see action potential and depolarization.*

Reproduction

The process by which offsprings are produced.

Residual Body

A secondary lysosome that contains indigestible wastes.

Resorption (bone)

The dissolution of bone calcium phosphate crystals by the action of osteoclasts. *Also see parathyroid hormone.*

Respiratory Acidosis

A decreased blood pH caused by an *increased* carbon dioxide tension (PCO_2). The CO_2 combines with H_2O to produce carbonic acid thus increasing acidity. It is almost always caused by alveolar *hypoventilation.*

Respiratory Alkalosis

An increased blood pH caused by a *decreased* arterial carbon dioxide tension (PCO_2). The most common cause is *hyperventilation* as may occur in states of severe anxiety and fear and during mechanical ventilation. Deliberate hyperventilation is sometimes used to lower intracranial pressure (ICP) because of the cerebral vasoconstricting effect of hypocapnia ($\downarrow PCO_2$). *Also see metabolic alkalosis.*

Respiratory burst

The release of reactive oxygen species from neutrophils and macrophages in response to the presence of foreign bodies.

Respiratory Distress Syndrome (RDS)

See Hyaline membrane disease.

Respiratory membrane

Lung membrane through which gas exchange occurs between the alveoli and the pulmonary blood. Also called pulmonary membrane.

Respiratory Quotient (RQ)

The ratio of CO_2 produced to O_2 consumed per unit time in the metabolism of the various classes of food. RQ for carbohydrates is 1.0; Fat = 0.7; Protein = 0.8. The reason for this is that one molecule of carbon dioxide is produced for every molecule of oxygen used to metabolize carbohydrates. Reaction of oxygen with fat produces a significant amount of water (and so less CO_2) due to the reaction of oxygen with hydrogen. Carbohydrates are the first to be metabolized immediately following a meal; therefore, RQ will be approximately 1. A few hours later, the carbohydrates are used up and RQ would approach 0.7. Thus, in conditions like severe and untreated diabetes mellitus in which carbohydrate metabolism is suppressed (due to a lack of insulin), RQ will tend towards 0.7. Whole body RQ on a normal diet is about 0.82.

Respiratory Zone

Portion of the lungs comprising the respiratory bronchioles and the terminal alveoli, where gas exchange with pulmonary blood occurs. *Also see conducting zone and dead space.*

Resting Potential

See membrane potential.

Reticular Activating System (RAS)

Part of the reticular formation situated between the brain stem and the cerebral cortex. It is involved in the sleep/wake cycle. The RAS is depressed during sleep.

Reticular formation

A complex network of fibers situated in the brain stem. It arouses the cerebral cortex, affects voluntary movement, and influences cardio-respiratory function.

Reticulocytes

Immature red blood cells that contain basophilic filaments; they constitute about 1% of the total red blood cells. An increased reticulocyte count is an indication of increased erythropoiesis.

Reticuloendothelial system (RES)

A component of the immune system that consists of phagocytic cells (macrophages, monocytes) and present in large numbers in lymph nodes and the spleen; the RES also includes Kupffer cells in the liver and specialized endothelial cells in lymphatic tissues and bone marrow fibroblasts.

Reticulospinal tract

Nerve fiber tracts that arise from the pontine and medullary reticular formation; fibers of the pontine reticulospinal tract exert facilitating control over voluntary movements. The medullary reticulospinal tract inhibits voluntary motor activities. Both fiber tracts receive input signals from the motor cortex.

Retina

The innermost layer of the eye; it contains neurons and photoreceptors (rods and cones).

Retinine

The chemical precursor of the photosensitive visual pigment, rhodopsin.

Reynold's number (Re)

A number that expresses the relationship of certain variables that predict the probability of laminar (streamline) or turbulent flow as fluid flows through a vessel or tube.

$Re = \varrho \upsilon d / \eta$

where ϱ = density

υ = linear velocity of the fluid

d = diameter of the tube or vessel

η = viscosity of the fluid

$Re > 2000$ is associated with turbulent flow and below that, flow is usually laminar. If all other variables are constant, the critical velocity is that at which Reynolds number reaches or exceeds 2000 and turbulent flow ensues. This principle has wide clinical applications in many situations where fluids flow through a vessel or tube.

Korotkoff sounds are the result of turbulent flow in the artery during auscultatory blood pressure measurement. Another common application of this principle is the use of a helium/oxygen mixture to lower the density of inspired gas in patients with stridor. This lowers the Reynolds number to below 2000 and allows laminar flow. *Osborne Reynolds, Irish-born English Engineer (1842-1912).*

Rhodopsin (Visual purple)

A light-sensitive photoreceptor protein (of the G-protein coupled receptor family). It consists of scotopsin and retinal (derived from vitamin A in the retina). Rhodopsin is responsible for monochromatic vision in the dark.

Riboflavin

Vitamin B_2 of the B complex family. A water-soluble micronutrient that is important for body growth, red blood cell formation, and energy release from carbohydrates.

Ribosome

A cytoplasmic organelle that is the site for protein synthesis; it is composed of protein and ribosomal RNA.

Rickets

A metabolic bone disease in children characterized by a failure of mineralization of growing bone and/or other osteoid tissue. It is caused by vitamin D deficiency from inadequate exposure to sunlight (necessary for vitamin D synthesis) or inadequate intake. Common in the tropics where infants are swaddled and women and infants may spend prolonged periods indoors. The same phenomenon in adult bone results in *osteomalacia. Also see 1,25-dihydroxycholecalciferol and parathyroid hormone.*

Rinne's Test

A test used to compare bone and air conduction by using the stem and tines of a vibrating tuning fork, respectively. *Also see Weber test, audiometry, and deafness.*

RNA (Ribonucleic Acid)

A nucleic acid that is composed of nitrogenous bases, ribose sugar and phosphate groups; there are three cytoplasmic forms: messenger RNA (mRNA) transfer RNA (tRNA) and ribosomal RNA (rRNA).

RNA polymerase

An enzyme that joins nucleotides complementary to a DNA template during the cellular process of transcription.

Rods

Visual photoreceptors in the retina that respond to dim light.

S

Saccadic Eye Movements	Conjugate and voluntary eye movements that enable the eyes to rapidly acquire objects and change fixation in the visual scene. This brings the retinal image onto the fovea.
Saccule	A membranous sac-like cavity that is located in the vestibule of the inner ear; it contains sensory receptors that are responsible for static equilibrium.
Salivary Glands	Glands responsible for the secretion of salivary juice; There are 3 main types (paired): parotid, submandibular (submaxillary) and sublingual glands. Parasympathetic stimulation produces excessive salivation. Anticholinergic agents such as glycopyrrolate and atropine reduce salivation (antisialologue effect). *Also see ptyalin, salivatory nuclei, and acetylcholine.*
Salivatory nuclei	Comprise the superior and inferior salivatory nuclei; they are located in the brain stem and they regulate secretion by salivary glands through a parasympathetic pathway. *Also see salivary glands.*
Saltatory Conduction	A characteristic mode of transmission of nerve impulse in myelinated axons in which action potentials are conducted rapidly from one node of Ranvier to another. *Also see nodes of Ranvier and myelin sheath.*
Sarcolemma	The plasma membrane of muscle fiber.
Sarcomere	The structural and functional subunit of a myofibril in striated muscle. It contains actin and myosin filaments and is the distance between two successive Z lines. Contraction results in muscle activity. *Also see actin and myosin.*
Sarcoplasm	The cytoplasm of striated muscle cells.
Sarcoplasmic Reticulum (SR)	Tubular network within a muscle fiber corresponding to the smooth endoplasmic reticulum of striated muscle cells. It surrounds each myofibril and is a major site for Ca^{2+} ions storage. The SR releases and sequesters Ca^{2+} during contraction and relaxation, respectively. Failure of Ca^{2+} sequestration results in prolonged contraction with no relaxation (contracture) and a hypermetabolic state. This is believed to be the molecular mechanism

of the rare life-threatening condition called *malignant hyperthermia* (MH). *Also see endoplasmic reticulum and hyperpyrexia.*

Satellite Cells

Also called ganglionic gliocytes. Cells in the peripheral nervous system which encapsulate dorsal root and cranial nerve ganglion cells; they have regulatory functions similar to astrocytes.

Satiety Center

Located in the hypothalamus, regulates feeding; electrical stimulation of this center in experimental animals stops the feeding behavior. *Also see food intake regulation.*

Satiety Factor

An appetite-reducing substance secreted into the circulation by adipose tissue. Secretion increases following a meal and decreases during fasting. *Also see food intake regulation.*

Schwann cells

A supporting (neuroglial) cell that spirally envelopes the fiber of a peripheral neuron forming the myelin sheath around the axon. Function is similar to oligodendrocytes in the CNS. Schwann cells also direct regeneration of peripheral nerve fibers to their target cells. Also called *Schwann's membrane or sheath of Schwann. Also see glial cell, myelin sheath, and nodes of Ranvier.*

Schizophrenia

A major psychiatric disorder characterized by disturbances in thought (delusions, hallucinations), perception, behavior and affect that is of a chronic and deteriorating nature. It affects 1% of the world's population and accounts for 20% of all psychiatric illnesses. Derived from the Greek words *schizo* (split, divide) and *phrenos* (mind).

Sclera

The tough white outer layer of the eyeball. It is composed of fibrin connective tissue.

Sclerotome

The part of the somite that gives rise to bone.

Scotopic Vision

Conditions of reduced lighting; most suited for operation of low-threshold photoreceptors (rods).

Scurvy

A condition arising from ascorbic acid (vitamin C) deficiency. Ascorbic acid is essential for collagen formation.

Sebaceous Glands

Exocrine glands in the skin that secrete oily sebum into hair follicles.

Sebum

Oily secretion produced by sebaceous glands; it provides lubrication for the cornified surface of the skin.

Secretagogue

A substance that causes the secretion of another substance. It acts by increasing the cellular levels of second messengers (Ca^{2+} or cAMP), which in turn stimulates a particular cell to secrete. Angiotensin II is an example of a secretagogue as it causes the adrenal glands to secrete aldosterone.

Secretin

A polypeptide hormone secreted by the mucosa of the small intestine in response to the presence of acid chyme in the intestine. It stimulates the release of bicarbonate-rich pancreatic juice and inhibits small intestinal motility.

Segmentation

A form of "segmental" movement that occurs in the small intestine; it ensures mixing of chyme with intestinal secretions.

Sella Turcica

A socket in the sphenoid bone in which the pituitary gland is located.

Semen

The thick, whitish fluid ejaculated by the penis; it consists of sperm and secretions from the prostate and seminal vesicles.

Semicircular Canals

Three tubular structures located within the inner ear; contains sensory receptors responsible for the sense of equilibrium.

Semilunar valves

Half-moon shaped heart valves; found in the aortic and pulmonary valves.

Seminal Vesicle

Accessory sex organ in males; has exocrine function and its secretions contain fructose, prostaglandins, LH, FSH, plasminogen activating factor, prolactin, testosterone and proteases.

Seminiferous tubules

The tubules within the testes in which spermatogenesis occurs.

Semipermeable membrane

A membrane with varying degrees of permeability; the size of the pores permits differential passage of solutes and other molecules and prevents the passage of others.

Sensory Neuron

An afferent neuron which typically possesses a long dendrite and short axon; it conducts nerve impulses from peripheral sensory organs into the central nervous system.

Series Elasticity

A common feature of contracting muscle due to the elastic nature of structural elements such as cross bridges of the muscle. The cross bridges lengthen when force is generated.

Serotonin

An autocoid and monoamine neurotransmitter. Known as 5-hydroxytryptamine (5HT), it is derived from the amino acid L-tryptophan and is present in platelets, enterochromaffin cells, and the brain. Various subtypes of serotonin receptors have been identified (5-HT$_1$, 5-HT$_2$, 5-HT$_3$ and 5-HT$_4$). Serotonin released at synapses in the brain has been associated with the regulation of mood and behavior, appetite, and the cerebral circulation. There is an abundance of 5HT$_3$ receptors in the area prostrema of the brain stem and these are believed to influence the emetic center. 5HT$_3$ receptor antagonists such as ondansetron and dolasetron are widely used for the prevention and treatment of nausea and vomiting. *Also see tryptophan.*

Serous membrane (Serosa)

Thin membranous lining of internal body cavity; it has two layers and the space between them is filled with serous fluid.

Sertoli Cells

Cells in the seminiferous tubules that support, nourish, and regulate the spermatogenic cells. *Also called sustentacular cells.*

Serum

The straw-colored liquid that remains after clotting of blood. Serum is plasma from which fibrinogen and other clotting factors have been removed. *Also see plasma.*

Sex Chromosomes

Unequal pairs of chromosomes (X and Y), which contain genes for sex determination (based on the presence or absence of a Y chromosome). Females lack a Y chromosome and have XX genotype. Males have a Y chromosome and have the XY genotype.

Sex Steroids

Androgens and estrogens; they are responsible for the development and maintenance of secondary sexual characteristics.

"Sham Rage"

Occurs following the surgical separation of the hypothalamus from higher centers. A "sham rage" animal displays emotional behavior similar to that of an enraged intact animal. Because of the emotional component associated with the "rage" response in experimental animals, some believe that this term should be dropped. Rage reactions may be seen in patients with brain injury from various causes and also following certain neurosurgical procedures.

Shock

A state of generalized circulatory insufficiency that is associated with a rapid decrease in cardiac output, decreased end organ perfusion and if untreated, can lead to multiple organ failure and death. Types of shock include: hypovolemic or hemorrhagic shock, cardiogenic shock, distributive (anaphylactic, septic, neurogenic) shock and obstructive (tension pneumothorax, cardiac tamponade) shock. Massive blood loss, especially associated with major trauma, is a common cause of shock. Four grades of shock have been described based on the percentage of blood or volume loss from the effective circulation:

Grade I:	≤15%
Grade II:	15-30%
Grade III:	30-40%
Grade IV:	>40%

Grade III marks the onset of decompensated shock (failure of compensatory mechanisms) and Class IV is immediately life-threatening since circulatory collapse is imminent.

Fluid and blood resuscitation, pharmacologic support, and treatment of the underlying cause are the key elements to the successful management of all types of shock.

Also see hypovolemic shock and cardiogenic shock.

Abnormal HR (Tachycardia, Bradycardia)

Low C.O → Low BP ← Low TPR

Low Venous Return
Low Stroke Volume
Low Blood Volume

Generalized Vasodilation

SHOCK

C.O = Cardiac output; HR = Heart Rate; BP = Blood Pressure
TPR = Total Peripheral Resistance

Mechanism of Shock

Sick Sinus Syndrome

An intrinsic disease of the sinoatrial node in which it is unable to function as the dominant pacemaker. The recovery time from overdrive suppression by an ectopic focus is greatly prolonged. Commonly associated with bradycardia and a combination of bradycardia and tachycardia (Tachy-Brady syndrome) and other arrhythmias. Cardiac pacing is the treatment of choice in severe cases. *Also see sinoatrial node.*

Sickle Cell Anemia (SCA)

An inherited hemoglobinopathy characterized by chronic hemolytic anemia and multiple end-organ damage. Although the disease was well known to Africans for hundreds of years, it was first described in western literature by a Chicago physician (Dr. James B. Herrick) in 1910 in an affluent dental student from the West Indies. It is caused by a mutation in the beta chain of the hemoglobin molecule resulting in a single amino acid substitution (valine for glutamic acid on position 6 from the amino end) and the formation of hemoglobin S. The mutant gene has been located on the short arm of chromosome 11. Homozygous inheritance results in (Hb SS) while heterozygous inheritance causes (Hb AS) or sickle cell trait. Five haplotypes of the mutant beta allele (four originating in Africa and one from the Persian gulf and Asia) have been identified and their importance relates to the amount of protective fetal hemoglobin present in adult patients with SCA. This may explain the difference in severity of SCA. Conventional teaching about the mechanism of organ damage in SCA relates to polymerization of hemoglobin S under conditions of low oxygen tension. This causes the red cells to become sickle-shaped, hemolyze, and clog up blood vessels, especially at the microcirculatory level. Current knowledge suggests that the most important mechanism responsible for the devastating effects of SCA is a disruption of nitric oxide (NO) transport from the lungs to the vascular endothelium due to the abnormal hemoglobin. This results in chronic endothelial inflammation, microvascular occlusion, end-organ vaso-occlusive infarction and major disability and death. It is most prevalent in West and Central Africa, parts of India, and in the southern Mediterranean. 10% of Blacks in the USA and UK have the sickle cell trait and 0.3% of blacks in the USA have sickle cell anemia. Sickle cell trait confers some protection against falciparum malaria and this seems to have allowed perpetuation of the abnormal gene. Definitive diagnosis is by hemoglobin electrophoresis. *Also see, anemia, fetal hemoglobin, and electrophoresis.*

SIF Cells

See small intensely fluorescent cells.

Single Unit Tissues

Excitable tissues such as the heart and smooth muscles lining tubular visceral organs; all the cells respond as a syncytium because of the presence of cell-to-cell contacts.

Sinoatrial Node (SA Node)

Specialized cardiac tissue located in the upper wall of the right atrium. Called the *pacemaker* because it initiates the normal heart beat. *Also see cardiac conduction system and sick sinus syndrome*

Sinusoids

Minute blood vessels that take the place of capillaries in certain organs such as the liver and bone-marrow. They are larger in diameter than capillaries.

Skeletal Muscle Pump

Skeletal muscle contraction that compresses the veins and enhances venous return.

Sleep

A state of unconsciousness from which an individual can be easily aroused by various stimuli. There are two types of sleep: slow wave sleep or non-rapid eye movement sleep (NREM) and rapid eye movement (REM) sleep (or paradoxical sleep). Dreams occurring during REM sleep are believed to be better remembered than those of slow wave sleep.

Sleep Apnea

See obstructive sleep apnea (OSA) and apnea.

Sliding Filament Theory

Describes the cellular process involving the movement of actin filaments in relation to myosin filaments to produce muscle contraction; the sarcomere shortens while the lengths of the filaments remain unchanged.

Slow-Reacting Substance of Anaphylaxis

See leukotrienes and eicosanoids.

Slow Waves

Low-frequency oscillations of the resting membrane potential of gastrointestinal smooth muscle.

Small Intensely Fluorescent (SIF) cells

Inhibitory inter-neurons found in some autonomic ganglia. They contain large amounts of catecholamines and are observable by fluorescent histochemistry.

Smooth Muscle

A non-striated involuntary muscle tissue found in the walls of internal organs; two subtypes exist: single unit and multi-unit.

Snellen's Chart

A chart utilized for the assessment of visual acuity.

Sodium-Potassium Pump

An active transport protein in the plasma membrane. By accumulating K^+ within cells and extruding Na^+ from cells, it maintains gradients for these ions across the cell membrane. *Also see ATPase.*

Somatesthetic Sensations

Sensations that arise from joint, cutaneous, muscle and tendon receptors; cortical perception occurs at the post-central gyrus.

Somatic Motor Neurons

Neurons that innervate skeletal muscle fibers; their cell bodies are located in the spinal cord or brain stem.

Somatomammotropin (Human Chorionic)

A hormone of pregnancy. Plasma levels of human chorionic somatomammotropin (hCS) are used as a marker for placental function. hCS also stimulates lipolysis and antagonizes the actions of insulin on carbohydrate metabolism. Also called *human placental lactogen (hPL)*

Somatomedin

Peptides which mediate the actions of growth hormone; they also enhance somatostatin synthesis and release. *Also See Insulin-like growth factors (IGFs).*

Somatostatin

A polypeptide hormone secreted by the hypothalamus and by the delta cells of the endocrine pancreas; it inhibits the secretion of growth hormone from the anterior pituitary.

Somatotropic Hormone

See Growth hormone.

Somites

Blocks of mesoderm arranged on either side of the embryonic neural tube. They differentiate into the sclerotome and the dermomyotome, which form the vertebral column and the segmental muscles, respectively.

Somnolence

A state of drowsiness or excessive sleepiness.

Sounds of Korotkoff

The sounds heard with a stethoscope during auscultatory blood pressure measurement; they are presumed to be caused by turbulent flow in a major vessel (brachial artery) that results from blood jetting through the partially occluded vessel. *Also see auscultatory blood pressure measurement and Reynold's number.*

Spastic Paralysis

Sustained state of skeletal muscle contracture due to inability to degrade acetylcholine released at the neuromuscular junction; it may be drug-induced or caused by spinal cord injury.

Spatial Summation

A process by which two separate (presynaptic) action potentials stimulate the postsynaptic cell in an additive fashion.

Spermatids

Cells formed in the seminiferous tubules by meiosis; on maturation, they become spermatozoa.

Spermatocytes

Cells arising from the modified and enlarged spermatogonia. They cross into the Sertoli cell layer and develop into primary spermatocytes. Meiotic division of the primary spermatocytes results in the secondary spematocytes. Secondary spermatocytes form spermatids.

Spermatogenesis

The formation of spermatozoa; it occurs in the seminiferous tubules and is stimulated by the anterior pituitary gonadotropic hormone.

Spermatogonia

Derived from primordial germ cells; they give rise to spermatozoa.

Spermatozoon

A mature sperm cell, derived from a spermatid.

Spermiogenesis

A process by which interconnected spermatids develop into separate mature spermatozoa. It is the final stage of spermatogenesis.

Sphincter

Ring of smooth muscle in the wall of a tubular or hollow organ; maintains tonic contraction that produces constriction. Examples include: pyloric sphincter and the upper and lower esophageal sphincters. Sphincters sometimes lack clear anatomic boundaries.

Sphingomyelin

A major type of sphingophospholipid found in cell membranes. A disorder of lipid metabolism with accumulation of sphingomyelin occurs in *Niemann-Pick disease.*

Sphygmomanometer

A blood pressure measuring device consisting of a pressure gauge and an inflatable cuff that wraps around an extremity. *Also see auscultatory blood pressure measurement.*

Spinal Reflex

A reflex that is coordinated at the level of the spinal cord. *Also see reflex.*

Spinal Shock

Shock resulting from transection of the spinal cord or acute spinal cord injury. Associated with flaccid paralysis, loss of autonomic functions and loss of all sensation below the level of transection or injury. Severe hypotension and bradycardia are features of a high spinal cord injury or transection.

Spinomesencephalic Tract

A somatosensory pathway of the ventral spinal cord with fibers terminating in several nuclei of the midbrain. Cells of this tract respond to noxious stimuli.

Spinothalamic Tract

A major sensory pathway for pain, thermal, and tactile sensations. There are two spinothalamic tracts: the *lateral* spinothalamic tract transmits pain, heat and cold sensations. The *anterior* spinothalamic tract transmits pressure and touch sensations. *Also see pain.*

Spiral Organ

See Organ of Corti.

Spirometer

A device used for the measurement of lung volumes and calculation of flow rates. Two types are described: *wet* spirometer (Benedict Roth) and a *dry* spirometer (Vitalograph).

Spirometry

The measurement of lung volumes and the calculation of flow rates using a spirometer. A type of pulmonary function test that provides information about obstructive or restrictive lung diseases. Useful for assessing the efficacy of bronchodilator therapy, especially in asthmatic patients. *Also see forced vital capacity.*

Spironolactone

A synthetic steroid diuretic that competitively blocks the actions of aldosterone. It increases the excretion of salt and water but conserves potassium, hence its classification as a *potassium-sparing* diuretic.

Splanchnic circulation

Circulation consisting of blood supply to the viscera (gastrointestinal tract, liver, spleen and pancreas).

Spleen

Mass of lymphoid tissue located in the abdominal cavity. A component of the reticuloendothelial system and is an important source of lymphocytes and a store for RBCs.

Sprue

A malabsorption syndrome characterized by nutritional deficiencies, flattened intestinal epithelium and decreased density of microvilli. Occurs in tropical and non-tropical forms. The tropical form is common in the Caribbean, Southeast Asia and parts of India. The non-tropical form is called *celiac disease* or *celiac sprue.*

Staircase Phenomenon (Treppe)

A progressive increase in the force of muscle contraction. It is due to a change in the frequency of contraction and is believed to be the result of increased intracellular Ca^{2+}. *"Treppe"* is the German term for *staircase.*

Starling forces

Describes the factors that determine fluid movement across the capillary wall. The capillary hydrostatic pressure and the interstitial fluid oncotic pressure encourage fluid movement into the interstitial space. This is opposed by the capillary oncotic pressure and the interstitial fluid hydrostatic pressure.

$$Q = K[(P_c - P_i) - \sigma (\pi_c - \pi_i)]$$

where Q = fluid flow

K = capillary filtration coefficient
P_c = capillary hydrostatic pressure
P_i = interstitial hydrostatic pressure
σ = reflection coefficient for plasma proteins by the endothelium
π_c = capillary oncotic pressure
π_i = interstitial oncotic pressure

Also see colloid osmotic pressure. Ernest Starling (1866-1927), English Physiologist.

Starling's law of the heart

See Frank-Starling law of the heart.

Steatorrhea

The presence of excessive amounts of fat in the stool resulting in bulky, pale, and foul-smelling feces. Seen commonly in malabsorption syndromes.

Stem Cells

See pluripotent cells.

Stercobilin

A product of bilirubin metabolism that is responsible for the brown coloration of stool. *Also see urobilin.*

Stereognosis

The ability to recognize the shape of objects placed in the hand; this sensation is lost following a lesion of the ascending pathway of the dorsal portion of the spinal cord.

Stereopsis

The perception of distance by binocular vision.

Steroid

Synthetic or naturally-occurring fat-soluble organic compound derived from cholesterol. Have significant anti-inflammatory and immunosuppressive effects. Used for replacement therapy in conditions of steroid deficiency and as an immunosuppressant. Other uses are largely empirical. Prolonged steroid therapy is associated with several untoward effects.

Stokes-Adams syndrome

Periodic fainting spells associated with complete atrioventricular block and resulting from cerebral hypoperfusion. An artificial pacemaker is the treatment of choice.

Streptokinase

A protein formed by some B-hemolytic streptococci; used clinically to dissolve clots especially in the setting of myocardial infarction and pulmonary embolism (thrombolytic therapy). Acts by conversion of plasminogen to plasmin. *Also see fibrinolysin and fibrinolysis.*

Stress

A physical or psychological stimulus that alters the body's physiological state; it is characterized by increased heart rate, a rise in arterial blood pressure, muscular tension, irritability and depression. The *stress response* refers to the various metabolic and neuroendocrine changes that occur after surgery, trauma, severe burns and other major physiologic insults.

Stretch Reflex

See myotatic reflex.

Striated Muscle

Muscle tissue (skeletal and cardiac) characterized by transverse striations.

Striosomes

Subdivisions of the striatum that contain projections of the limbic system; striosomes are presumed to modulate the dopaminergic nigrostriatal pathway.

Stroke Volume (SV)

The volume of blood pumped by each ventricle with each heart beat. Cardiac output is the product of SV and heart rate. Also expressed as end diastolic volume (EDV) – end systolic volume (ESV).

Strychnine

A poison obtained from seeds of a tree native to the Asian sub-region. It acts by blocking glycine receptor proteins producing spastic paralysis. Although no longer in clinical use, it is used in certain rat poisons and is mixed with certain street drugs.

Stuart Factor

Factor X of the clotting process; secreted by hepatocytes.

Subarachnoid space

The space between the pia mater and arachnoid; it contains cerebrospinal fluid (CSF). The lumbar subarachnoid space is frequently utilized to obtain a CSF sample (lumbar puncture) and also for performance of subarachnoid block (spinal) for certain surgical procedures. Also called the intrathecal space.

Sublingual Gland

See salivary glands.

Submucosal plexus

A neuronal plexus of the enteric nervous system, located in the submucosa; it is also called Meissner's plexus.

Substance P

An eleven-amino acid neuropeptide neurotransmitter found in the brain, spinal cord, and enteric neurons of the gastrointestinal tract. It plays an important role in pain transmission and inflammatory processes.

Substrate

A molecule that combines with the active sites of an enzyme and is acted upon by the catalytic action of the enzyme.

Sudden Infant Death Syndrome (SIDS)

The sudden death of an infant that is unexpected and unexplained by a thorough postmortem investigation to include: an autopsy and a detailed examination of the scene. Called cot death in most Commonwealth countries and crib death in North America. Several risk factors have been identified but the exact cause remains unknown. Recent studies suggest the possible role of serotonin and certain bacterial infections in the etiology of SIDS.

Sulcus

A deep groove or furrow in the cerebral cortex that separates the gyri of the cerebral cortex. *Also see gyrus.*

Summation

Additive effects (in neurons) of graded synaptic potentials; it also denotes additive effects of contractile responses of different muscle fibers.

Superior colliculus

A layered structure comprising superficial and deeper layers that serves as a center for visual reflexes.

Suppressor T Cells

A subpopulation of T lymphocytes. They suppress the immune response of other lymphocytes, thus preventing the destruction of normal tissue.

Suprachiasmatic nucleus (SCN)

A nucleus located above the optic chiasm in the hypothalamus. Its primary function is the regulation of circadian rhythms. Through neuronal signals to other hypothalamic nuclei and the pineal gland, the SCN modulates body temperature and the release of cortisol and melatonin.

Supraoptic nucleus

Located in the hypothalamus and contains neurons that produce ADH and oxytocin.

Surfactant

An amphipathic lipoprotein compound secreted by pulmonary alveoli cells; it stabilizes pulmonary tissue by reducing surface tension in the alveoli. *Also see pneumocytes and hyaline membrane disease.*

Swallowing

See deglutition

Sympathetic Nervous System (SNS)

A division of the autonomic nervous system. Sympathetic neurons have short preganglionic fibers that terminate on the sympathetic chain (paravertebral ganglia) along both sides of the vertebral column. The ganglia are located close to the CNS, in contrast to those of the parasympathetic nervous system that are located close to/or within effector organs. Some preganglionic fibers synapse in collateral (prevertebral) ganglia: the celiac, superior and inferior mesenteric ganglia. Some preganglionic fibers synapse directly with the adrenal medulla, which upon stimulation, releases epinephrine and some norepinephrine into the circulation. Sympathetic nerves originate in the spinal cord between the thoracic (T1) and lumbar (L2) regions; hence the SNS is often called the "thoraco-lumbar" outflow.

Sympathetic Tone

A state of continuous sympathetic discharge that prepares the body for the "flight or fight" response; it is associated with:

- Increased release of catecholamines by the adrenal medulla
- Increased heart rate
- Increased cardiac contractility
- Increase in arterial blood pressure
- Decreased blood flow to visceral organs
- Increased skeletal muscle blood flow
- Bronchodilation
- Renal retention of sodium and water

Central neuraxial blocks (epidural and spinal) and high spinal cord injuries can produce marked ablation of sympathetic tone that can result in profound hypotension unless fluid resuscitation is administered. Pharmacologic support may also be required.

Symport

A form of membrane transport in which two dissimilar molecules or ions move in the same direction by means of a common carrier mechanism.

Synapse

A region of close proximity between an axon bulb and the dendrite (cell body) of another neuron. The two main types of synapses are: chemical synapse and electrical synapse. *Chemical synapses:* The presynaptic neuron secretes neurotransmitter substances (e.g. acetylcholine, noradrenaline, histamine, serotonin, and glycine), which diffuse across the synaptic cleft, to stimulate receptors located on the postsynaptic neuronal membrane.

Electrical synapses: Involve the transport of ions and the spread of action potentials through gap junctions, particularly in visceral smooth muscle and cardiac muscle cells.

Synapsin

A protein that regulates neurotransmitter release at neuronal synapses. It acts by altering the number of synaptic vesicles available for release by exocytosis.

Synaptic Cleft

The region between two neurons or a neuron and an effector organ across which neurotransmitter substances diffuse in response to the presynaptic action potential.

Synaptic Plasticity

The ability of neurons to form new synaptic associations; it also denotes the ability of a presynaptic neuron to release more than one type of neurotransmitter.

Synaptosome

Sac-like artificial vesicles obtained after homogenization and fractionation of neural tissue; it is also called an "isolated synapse." It comprises vesicles and mitochondria.

Syncope (Fainting)

A sudden and temporary loss of consciousness. Caused by a decreased cerebral blood flow secondary to a decreased cardiac output. Usually of cardiovascular etiology such as arrhythmias, conduction anomalies and heart block. Fixed cardiac output states such as aortic stenosis may cause exertional syncope. Common non-cardiovascular causes include hyperventilation (hypocapnia) and hypoglycemia.

Syncytium (Functional)

A term denoting a single functioning unit such as the myocardium and gastrointestinal smooth muscle. Action potentials originating in any of the cells can be transmitted to all the other cells.

Synergism

A phenomenon where the combined effect of two similar drugs, hormones or regulatory processes exceeds an algebraic summation of the two agents or processes.

Systemic Circulation

The circuit of circulation that delivers blood to all parts of the body except the lungs; oxygenated blood from the left ventricle circulates through the arteries and capillaries to the tissues while deoxygenated (venous) blood is carried by veins to the right atrium. *Also see pulmonary circulation.*

Systemic vascular resistance (SVR)

See total peripheral resistance (TPR) and appendix I

Systole

The contraction phase of the cardiac cycle during which blood is pumped from the ventricles to the aorta and pulmonary artery. *Also see diastole.*

T

Tachycardia
An increased heart rate, usually greater than 100 beats per minute in adults. May be part of a normal physiologic response e.g. exercise, pain, stress or may be pathologic such as fever, certain drugs, endocrine disorders and cardiac arrhythmias.

Tamoxifen
A synthetic compound that binds to estrogen receptors. It inhibits the growth of estrogen-responsive breast cancer.

Tanacytes
Pituitary cells that aid the transfer of regulatory substances from the cerebrospinal fluid to the pituitary.

Taste
The chemical sense consisting of four basic qualities: sweet, sour, bitter or salty. Also called gustation.

T Cells
Thymus-dependent lymphocytes. They are involved in cell-mediated immunity. *Also see lymphocytes, delayed hypersensitivity.*

T-Tubule
A myoplasmic compartment found in close association with the sarcoplasmic reticulum; serves as a storage site for calcium ions.

T-type Channels
Subtype of calcium channels; activated at more negative potentials than L-types channels. They are insensitive to normal Ca^{2+} channel blocking drugs but blocked by nickel ions (Ni^{2+}). *Also see L-type channels and calcium channel blockers.*

T-Wave
Present in a normal electrocardiogram; it denotes ventricular repolarization. *Also see ECG.*

Tear Glands
See lacrimal glands.

Telencephalon
One of the five secondary vesicles that forms the two large cerebral hemispheres. Includes the diencephalon, midbrain and parts of the hindbrain.

Telomeres
Locations at ends of chromosomes in which there is a loss of DNA sequences resulting in decreased ability of cells to replicate. They are presumed to be an indicator of senescence (aging). Because of their involvement with cell replication and aging, telomeres and the enzyme telomerase are potential targets for anti-cancer drug development.

Telophase

Terminal step of mitosis and the last step of the second meiotic division; nuclei revert to the resting stage. *Also see meiosis and mitosis.*

Temporal Lobe

The part of the cerebral cortex that is involved with the interpretation and association of auditory and visual information.

Temporal Summation

A process in which two or more action potentials in a single presynaptic neuron induce a stepwise increase in the postsynaptic potential.

Tendon

A dense connective tissue consisting almost entirely of parallel collagen fibers. It attaches muscles at the sites of their origin and insertion.

Teratogen

An agent or factor that produces a defect or defects in the developing embryo. Examples are infectious agents (rubella, HIV, CMV), physical agents (X-rays), chemical agents (thalidomide, alcohol, and certain hormones) and certain coexisting diseases such as maternal diabetes. *Also see thalidomide.*

Terminal bouton

Ending of a presynaptic cell at a synaptic cleft or effector cells.

Terminal cisternae

Enlarged portions of the sarcoplasmic reticulum where large amounts of Ca^{2+} ions are stored in a resting muscle fiber.

Testis

The paired male gonads that are located in the scrotum; they produce sperm and testosterone. Also called *testicles.*

Testis-Determining Factor

Denotes the gene that results in maleness during embryonic development. The testis-determining factor causes the male sex organs to develop; in its absence, the embryo develops as a female.

Testosterone

The major androgenic steroid hormone secreted by the interstitial cells of the testes after puberty.

Tetanus

A smooth sustained contraction of a muscle (as opposed to muscle twitching); it is usually induced by rapidly repeating stimuli. Tetanic stimulation is one of the modalities used in the assessment of neuromuscular function.

Tetany

A state of increased nerve and skeletal muscle excitability resulting from a low ionized calcium level. Associated with parathyroid hormone insufficiency and alkalosis.

Tetraiodothyronine (T$_4$)

The major hormone secreted by the thyroid gland; it contains four iodine atoms. T4 regulates metabolism by controlling the rate of oxidation in cells and stimulation of protein synthesis in many organs. A deficiency of this hormone in early childhood causes cretinism. Also called thyroxine, it is composed of 65% iodine.

Tetralogy of Fallot

A cyanotic congenital heart lesion characterized by the presence of a complex shunt (shunt and obstruction). Characteristic features include:

- A large malaligned ventricular septal defect (VSD)
- An overriding aorta that receives blood from both ventricles.
- Infundibular pulmonary stenosis
- Right ventricular hypertrophy

It occurs in about 10 per 10,000 births. Some variants may be acyanotic ("Pink Tet"). Surgical correction is usually required.

Tetrodotoxin

A toxin derived from the puffer fish and some amphibians; it blocks Na$^+$ channels and is employed to distinguish between neurally and non-neurally mediated mechanisms.

Thalamus

Part of the brain consisting of two masses of gray matter, located in the lateral walls of the third ventricle; an important center for integration of sensory impulses and is also involved in the arousal of the cerebral cortex.

Thalassemia

A hereditary hemoglobin disorder characterized by a deficiency in the synthesis or absence of the α or β chains of hemoglobin. Alpha thalassemia is prevalent in people of west African descent whilst the beta form is present primarily in people of Mediterranean origin. *Also see sickle cell anemia.*

Thalidomide

A mild tranquilizer. It was used to treat morning sickness in pregnant women in the late 1950s and early 1960s. It was soon found to cause severe birth defects (deformed or absent limbs) in babies born to mothers who had used the drug resulting in a worldwide ban. The L-isomer is now known to possess the tranquilizing properties whereas the D-isomer impairs fetal development and causes birth defects. More recently, thalidomide has seen some resurgence in the treatment of leprosy, multiple myeloma, and certain complications of AIDS. These indications remain controversial. It however remains banned in pregnant women and its overall global use remains very tightly regulated. *Also see teratogen.*

Thebesian vessels

Small-sized veins that connect capillary beds directly with cardiac chambers; also provide communication with cardiac veins.

Theca Cells

Cells that are developed around granulosa cells prior to ovulation and contribute to secretion of ovarian hormones (estrogens and progesterone).

Theophylline

A crystalline drug found in certain tea leaves; used for the treatment of asthma. Its bronchodilating actions are due to phosphodiesterase inhibition and increased levels of the second messenger – cAMP. *Also see cAMP, adenylyl cyclase and phosphodiesterase.*

Thermogenesis

Heat production by the body through mechanisms such as increased metabolic rate or shivering. Non-shivering thermogenesis occurs in infants and small children by burning of brown fat, located between the shoulder blades.

Thermoreceptors

Mechanoreceptors that detect changes in temperature.

Theta Waves

Low frequency waves (3-7 Hz), which occur interspersed with alpha waves, in stage 1 of slow wave sleep.

Thiamine

Also called vitamin B_1; a water-soluble vitamin. Absorption of thiamine is by Na^+-dependent active transport. Acts as a coenzyme in carbohydrate metabolism and is involved in nerve cell and myocardial function. Deficiency causes *beriberi* with neurologic and cardiovascular involvement.

Thick Filaments

Dark striations of myofibrils constituting the A-band in muscles; it contains the contractile protein, myosin. *Also see A band and myosin.*

Thin Filaments

The light or I-band of the myofibrils; contains the contractile protein, actin. *Also see actin, myosin, and intermediate filaments.*

Third ventricle

A narrow slit-like cavity located between the two thalami and connected to the lateral ventricles and the fourth ventricle. This constitutes the ventricular and cerebrospinal fluid circulatory system in the brain. Obstruction of this system results in hydrocephalus and a raised intracranial pressure. Surgical intervention (*shunting*) is often required.

Thoracic duct

The major lymphatic vessel that drains lymph from the abdomen and the lower limbs into the left brachiocephalic vein. Damage to or blockage of the thoracic duct during surgery or following trauma can result in chylous ascites or pleural effusion (*chylothorax*).

Thorax

Part of the body cavity that lies between the neck (inlet) and the diaphragm; the chest.

Threonine

An essential amino acid.

Threshold Stimulus

The minimum stimulus that is capable of producing an action potential in an excitable cell.

Thrombin

A serine protease involved in the hemostatic and fibrinolytic processes. Formed from circulating prothrombin, it converts fibrinogen to fibrin. *Also see prothrombin, fibrinolysis and fibrinolysin.*

Thrombocyte (platelet)

See platelet.

Thrombocytopenia

A decrease in the number of circulating platelets (thrombocytes). Mechanisms include: decreased production, splenic sequestration, destruction by macrophages, increased destruction, and dilutional (massive blood transfusion). Spontaneous bleeding can occur in severe cases.

Thrombomodulin

A cofactor present on the surface of endothelial cells. It binds thrombin to the cell surface.

Thrombopoietin

A glycoprotein hormone; it regulates the production of platelets from megakaryocytes in the bone marrow.

Thrombosis

The development or presence of a blood clot in the circulatory system. Blockage of a major vessel can result in ischemia or infarction. A major cause of cardiovascular (heart attacks) and neurologic (strokes) disease. Deep venous thrombosis is a major risk after trauma and certain surgical procedures. *Also see embolus.*

Thrombospondin

A protein synthesized by platelets, fibroblasts, monocytes, smooth muscle and endothelial cells; it is presumed to play a role in cell-to-cell adhesion.

Thromboxane

Produced from arachidonic acid in the cyclooxygenase pathway. It is the most potent platelet aggregator and also causes profound vasoconstriction. *Also see cyclooxygenase and non-steroidal anti-inflammatory drugs (NSAIDS).*

Thrombus

An abnormal clot in a blood vessel; produced by the formation of fibrin threads around a platelet plug.

Thymopoietin

A hormone secreted by the thymus gland. It exists in two forms: Thymopoietin I and II.

Thymosin

A hormone secreted by the thymus that promotes maturation of T-lymphocytes.

Thymus

A pinkish-grey lymphoid organ located along the trachea behind the sternum in the upper thoracic cavity. Its main function is to regulate the immune system. A poorly developed thymus in fetal life results in depressed T-cell immunodeficiency as is the case in DiGeorge syndrome. An enlarged thymus is seen in some patients with myasthenia gravis. *Also see cell mediated immunity, and myasthenia gravis.*

Thyroglobulin

A glycoprotein that is stored in the colloid of the thyroid follicles; it is a precursor for the iodine-containing thyroid hormones.

Thyroiditis

An inflammation of the thyroid gland. Chronic lymphocytic thyroiditis (Hashimoto's thyroiditis) is an autoimmune thyroiditis and is the most common cause of primary hypothyroidism. May also be of viral etiology.

Thyroid Releasing Hormone

A hormone produced by the hypothalamus; it stimulates the anterior pituitary to release thyroid-stimulating hormone (TSH).

Thyroid Stimulating Hormone (TSH)

Also called thyrotropin; it is a glycoprotein hormone secreted by the anterior pituitary gland; it stimulates the secretion of thyroxine and triiodothyronine by the thyroid gland.

Thyrotoxicosis

Hyperthyroidism; symptoms include nervousness, high state of excitability, muscular weakness, increased sweating, mild to extreme weight loss, fatigue with insomnia and heat intolerance. *Also see hyperthyroidism and Graves' disease.*

Thyroxine

See tetraiodothyronine (T_4).

Thyroxine-Binding Globulin

The major binding protein for the thyroid hormones, T4 and T3; it is synthesized in the liver.

Tidal Volume (V_T)

The amount of air or gas that is inspired and expired with each breath during quiet breathing. It is about 500mL in an adult or 7mL/Kg. The "actual" tidal volume is the tidal volume minus the anatomic dead space volume. *Also see dead space.*

Tight Junctions

Cell-to-cell contacts in which adjacent cell membrane proteins fuse to form an impregnable barrier. In the gastrointestinal tract, tight junctions are loose in the duodenum and tightest in the colon.

Tinnitus

A persistent ringing sound in the ears that occurs in the absence of a normal acoustic stimulus. May be caused by diseases of the ear, infections, brain tumors, Ménière's disease and ototoxcity from certain drugs (quinine, certain antibiotics). Other causes include pathological conditions of the inner ear or the auditory nerve; it is an early symptom of inner ear disease. *Also see Ménière's disease and vertigo.*

Tissue fluid

Part of the extracellular fluid that bathes the cells within body organs.

Tissue Plasminogen Activator (t-PA)

Serine proteases that convert plasminogen to plasmin; they are commonly employed to dissolve thrombi, especially in coronary arteries (thrombolytic therapy). *Also see fibrinolysin, fibrinolysis, streptokinase and urokinase.*

Tolerance

The gradual decrease in response to a drug following chronic exposure to the drug. May also occur following exposure to a related drug (*cross-tolerance*). Rapid development of tolerance is called *tachyphylaxis.* Possible mechanisms include receptor down-regulation and enzyme induction. Opioids, like morphine and related drugs, are examples of agents that produce tolerance.

Tone (Muscle)

A state of continuous partial contraction of muscle; it is necessary for the maintenance of posture.

Tonic Neck Reflexes

Positional reflexes; they are activated by the muscle spindles located in the neck muscles.

Tonic Stretch Reflex

The stretch reflex that is elicited by both the primary and secondary endings of muscle spindles.

Total Minute Volume

The product of tidal volume and respiratory rate. It is about 6 L/ minute in an adult.

Total Peripheral Resistance (TPR)

The sum of all the vascular resistances within the systemic circulation; it denotes resistance to blood flow in arteries and the resistance against which the heart pumps. TPR can be measured using the equation for blood flow:

R = DP/Q; where

R= resistance (mm Hg/ml/min),
DP = pressure difference (mm Hg) between the aorta and the vena cava
Q = Flow (ml/min): cardiac output.

In clinical practice it is expressed as:

[MAP – CVP (mm Hg) / CO (l/min)] x 80

Where, MAP is mean arterial pressure, CVP is central venous pressure, CO is cardiac output and 80 is a correction factor. Measurement requires the placement of a Swan-Ganz (pulmonary artery) catheter. TPR is also called the systemic vascular resistance (SVR). *Also see Appendix I.*

Totipotent stem cells

Primitive cells derived from embryonic yolk sac cells in the liver, spleen, and bone marrow. They are capable of differentiating into any cell type. *Also see pluripotent stem cell.*

Toxin

A poisonous substance capable of causing tissue injury or disease when introduced into the body; it can also act as an antigen and stimulate antibody production.

Trabeculae

A supporting framework of fibers that traverse the substance of a structure; e.g. the lamellae of spongy bone.

Tracts

A collection of nerve fibers within the central nervous system; it forms the white mater of the CNS.

Transamination

The process by which an amino group is transferred from an amino acid to an alpha-keto acid. It results in the formation of a new keto acid and a new amino acid without the appearance of free ammonia.

Transcortin

A specific corticosteroid-binding α-globulin (CBG) that binds plasma cortisol; the transcortin-cortisol complex is presumed to activate cellular adenylyl cyclase.

Transcription

The process by which the DNA sequence in a gene is copied into mRNA. *Also see translation.*

Transducer

Any device that converts one form of energy to another. The second form of energy is usually electrical. Transducers are widely used in measurement and monitoring devices/systems and have extensive laboratory and clinical applications.

Transducins

Regulatory G-proteins involved in vision; when light causes the photo-dissociation of rhodopsin, the G-protein alpha subunits dissociate from opsin and indirectly cause a reduction in the photoreceptor dark current.

Transferrin

A carrier protein that binds iron in the ferric state and transports it to the cells requiring it for heme synthesis. *Also see ferritin.*

Translation

The genetic process by which a protein molecule is synthesized from amino acids through the action of mRNA, tRNA, and ribosomes. The specificity of this process is under the control of the base sequences of the mRNA. *Also see transcription.*

Transplantation

The process by which tissue is grafted from one part of the body to another part or from a donor to a recipient.

Transpulmonary pressure

It is the difference between intrapulmonary (alveolar) pressure and the pleural pressure.

Treppe

See staircase phenomenon.

Trichromacy theory

A theory of color vision based on stimulation of three types of cones: red, green, and blue.

Tricuspid valve

The atrioventricular valve located between the right atrium and the right ventricle.

Trigone	The part of the urinary bladder that is between the ureteric openings and the urethra.
Triiodothyronine (T$_3$)	A hormone secreted by the thyroid gland; it is formed from thyroxine and is the physiologically active hormone in target cells. *Also see tetraiodothyronine (T$_4$).*
Tripeptide	Three amino acids bound together.
Triple response	A physiologic response that demonstrates the early phases of acute inflammation. It can be elicited by mechanical damage such as scratching a patch of skin. There is an initial *erythema* due to capillary dilatation followed by local swelling (*wheal*) due to increased permeability. Spread of the redness to the surrounding area is the *flare* and is due to arteriolar dilatation. Histamine release is an important factor in this response.
Tristearin	A triglyceride of stearic acid; a saturated fat that is the primary fat in beef.
Tritanopia	A form of color blindness associated with loss of the short wavelength system.
Trophic hormones	Hormones secreted by the anterior pituitary; names of the hormones end in the suffix – "tropin" e.g. corticotropin, thyrotropin, luteotropin. *Also see adenohypophysis.*
Trophoblast cells	Cells that give rise to the chorion and ultimately, form part of the placenta.
Tropomyosin	A filamentous muscle protein that attaches to actin; it acts together with troponin to inhibit and regulate the attachment of myosin cross bridges to actin. *Also see actin and myosin.*
Troponin	A muscle protein located in the thin filament of the sarcomeres of skeletal muscle; it is made up of three subunits: Troponin T, Troponin C and Troponin I. Cardiac troponin-I (TnI) is a biomarker, along with the clinical assessment and other tests, for the diagnosis of acute myocardial infarction.
Trypsin	A proteolytic enzyme secreted in pancreatic juice; it produces its digestive functions in the small intestine.
Tryptophan	An amino acid and precursor of niacin. It occurs in proteins and is essential for growth and normal body

metabolism. Deficiency can cause pellagra. It is also the precursor of the neurotransmitter serotonin. *Also see niacin and serotonin.*

TSH (Thyroid-Stimulating Hormone)

Also called *thyrotropin.* A glycoprotein hormone produced by the anterior pituitary and released to the circulation in a pulsatile manner. It stimulates thyroid functions using specific membrane G- protein coupled TSH receptors.

Tubocurarine

A non-depolarizing neuromuscular blocking drug derived from South American plants (*Chondrodendron tomentosum and Strychnos*). Used by native Indians as an arrow poison in the 16th century. Used in the treatment of tetanus in the late 1800. First used for muscle relaxation during anesthesia in 1942. Profound hypotension from sympathetic ganglia blockade is a common side effect with the use of this agent and may be beneficial in certain situations. More recently, its use has been surpassed by newer muscle relaxants especially in developed countries but it is still available as a useful agent in some developing countries. *Also see acetylcholine and acetylcholinesterase.*

Tubuloglomerular feedback

A negative feedback mechanism in which an increase in salt concentration or increased flow of filtrate at the distal tubule is sensed by the macula densa cells. The cells release a mediator that is transmitted to the glomerular microvasculature causing a constriction of the afferent arteriole.

Tumor Necrosis Factor (TNF)

An inflammation-promoting cytokine that is produced by monocytes and macrophages; it is effective in killing cancer cells. It is also secreted by adipose cells. Anti-TNF drugs have been developed for treatment of certain chronic inflammatory diseases such as Rheumatoid Arthritis.

Tunica albuginea

A tough, fibrous tissue surrounding the testis.

Turner's syndrome

A congenital abnormality in which one of the two X chromosomes is absent. They have a 45, X karyotype and usually have poorly developed gonads. Many newborns present with lymphedema and may also have cardiac abnormalities. A short, webbed neck and short stature are seen in the older child. Many variants exist and some patients appear normal and may be fertile.

Twitch (Muscle)

A rapid sequence of contraction and relaxation of a muscle fiber or a group of muscle fibers. Modifications of the twitch response are used for neuromuscular monitoring when muscle relaxants are used during anesthesia.

Tympanic Membrane

The eardrum; a thin membrane separating the inner part of the external auditory canal from the middle ear. It receives sound impulses from the outer ear and transmits them to the auditory ossicles. It also serves as the lateral wall of the tympanic cavity, separating it from the external auditory canal.

Tyrosine

A nonessential amino acid and the precursor of catecholamines.

Tyrosine kinase

An enzyme that adds a phosphate group to a tyrosine residue in a protein. In general, growth hormones and factors that promote cell division such as epidermal-derived growth factor and insulin-like growth factor act on tyrosine kinase receptors.

U

Ubiquinone	Part of the electron transport chain of the electron acceptors found on the inner mitochondrial membrane. It is also called Coenzyme-Q10.
Ulcer (Peptic)	*See peptic ulcer.*
Ultrafiltrate (glomerular)	*See glomerular ultrafiltrate.*
Universal Donor	*See ABO system.*
Universal Recipient	*See ABO system.*
Upper Esophageal Sphincter (UES)	Also called pharyngoesophageal sphincter; it consists of the cricopharyngeus muscle and the lower fibers of the inferior pharyngeal constrictor. It serves to prevent entry of air into the esophagus (aerophagia). *Also see lower esophageal sphincter (LES).*
Upper Motor Neuron (UMN)	First order neurons arising from the motor area of the cerebral cortex and extending to motor nuclei in the brain stem or the anterior horn cells of the spinal cord. *Also see lower motor neuron and motor neuron disease.*
Urea	A water-soluble compound and chief nitrogenous waste product of protein metabolism; produced from amino acids in the liver and excreted in the urine.
Uremia	The accumulation of nitrogen-containing waste products (urea) in blood; also called *azotemia.* Seen in renal failure. *Also see renal failure and azotemia.*
Ureter	Tubular structure that transports urine from the renal pelvis to the urinary bladder.
Urethra	Tubular structure that transports urine from the urinary bladder to the exterior. *Also see micturition.*
Uric Acid	Non-protein constituent of serum; formed in the liver by the breakdown of purines and excreted in the urine. Excessive accumulation results in deposition of uric acid crystals in the joints causing recurrent arthritis called gout.
Urine	Amber-colored metabolic waste fluid produced by the kidneys.
Urobilin	A breakdown product derived from bacterial degradation

of bilirubin; it contributes to the brownish coloration of feces. Present in small amounts in the urine. *Also see stercobilin.*

Urobilinogen

A product of bilirubin breakdown and a precursor for urobilin, formed in the intestine. Some urobilinogen is excreted in the feces and some is absorbed into the enterohepatic circulation.

Urokinase

A serine protease enzyme which converts plasminogen to plasmin; it is employed clinically for the dissolution of thrombi and emboli (thrombolytic therapy). *Also see fibrinolysin, fibrinolysis and streptokinase and tissue plasminogen activator.*

Urticaria

A skin reaction, usually of immunogenic etiology, producing redness and swelling of the skin. An anaphylactic reaction limited to the skin. A giant urticaria is sometimes called *angioedema* and it is an important cause of respiratory distress if the airway is affected.

Uterus

The womb; muscular structure in which the embryo develops.

Utricle

See Otolith organs.

V

Vaccination

Originally described in reference to active immunity. Now used in reference to any type of immunization. *Also see immunization.*

Vagina

The tubular genital canal in the female leading from the external opening (vulva) to the cervix.

Vagus nerve

The tenth cranial nerve; it is a mixed nerve (has both motor and sensory fibers) and is the major parasympathetic nerve in the body. It controls a wide variety of physiologic actions including: heart rate, gastrointestinal secretions and motility, sweating and speech. One of its branches, the recurrent laryngeal nerve, supplies the larynx. Derives its name from the Latin word for "wandering" because of its wide distribution.

Vagusstoff

See Acetylcholine.

Valsalva maneuver

Expiratory effort against a closed glottis; increases intrathoracic pressure, produces venoconstriction, and reduction in venous return. The cardiovascular compensatory mechanisms observed during this maneuver make it a useful test of the integrity of the autonomic nervous system.

Vasa recta

Capillaries that supply the medulla and papilla of the kidney.

Vasa vasorum

Blood vessel that supplies the walls of large blood vessel.

Vasectomy

A sterilization procedure that involves surgical removal of a portion of the vas deferens.

Vasoconstriction

A reduction in the diameter of blood vessels due to contraction of the smooth muscles in their walls.

Vasodilation

An increase in the diameter of blood vessels due to relaxation of the smooth muscles in their walls.

Vasomotor center

A center located in the reticular substance of the medulla and the lower third of the pons; it transmits autonomic signals to the heart (parasympathetic) and blood vessels (sympathetic). The three main components of the vasomotor center are: vasoconstrictor area, vasodilator area, and sensory area. The vasomotor center provides continuous sympathetic vasoconstrictor signals to blood vessels (vasomotor tone).

Vasopressin

See antidiuretic hormone (ADH).

Vein

A blood vessel that returns blood to the heart.

Venous Return

The return of deoxygenated blood from the veins to the heart. *Also see preload and central venous pressure.*

Venous Tone

The state of continuous constriction of veins; changes in venous tone affect both preload and circulating blood volume. *Also see preload and central venous pressure.*

Ventilation

Breathing; the process of moving air into and out of the lungs. *Also see artificial respiration.*

Ventilation-Perfusion Ratio (V/Q)

The ratio of alveolar ventilation to pulmonary blood flow; this ratio is important in the matching of alveolar ventilation to perfusion and provides for ideal gas exchange. Variation in V/Q ratio occurs in different parts of the lung but it averages 0.8. An increase in V/Q ratio is associated with increased dead space whilst a decrease ratio is associated with shunting. V/Q abnormalities are an important cause of hypoxemia in different lung diseases and altered physiologic states. Measurement of V/Q ratio by radioisotope techniques can aid the diagnosis of pulmonary embolism.

Ventricles

The two lower chambers of the heart. They receive blood from the atria and pump it into the systemic and pulmonary circulations.

Ventricular escape

Occurs when a ventricular focus initiates depolarization in place of the normal pacemaker (sinoatrial node); the resulting heart rhythm is termed *idioventricular*, and is characterized by a wide and bizarre QRS complex and absent P waves on the electrocardiogram.

Ventricular fibrillation

See fibrillation.

Ventrobasal complex

A relay nucleus located in the thalamus.

Venules

The smallest veins in the circulatory system; they connect capillaries to larger veins.

Vertigo

A false sensation of rotation associated with problems

with balance or gait. Causes are multi-factorial but ultimately result from vestibular system dysfunction. *Also see Ménière's disease and tinnitus.*

Vesicointestinal reflex

Inhibition of intestinal activity following urinary bladder irritation.

Vestibular system

The sensory system consisting of the semicircular canals and the Otolith organs. It maintains balance by detecting rotational movements and linear translations of the head. Neural signals for the vestibular system also control eye movement and muscles (for maintenance of posture). *Also see otolith organs.*

Vestibulo-ocular reflex

Compensatory eye movements resulting from rapid head movement; it involves transmission of signals from the semicircular canals directly to the eye muscles.

Villi

Finger-like projections of the small intestinal mucosa. They increase the absorptive surface of the intestines.

Viscera

The organs located within the abdominal or thoracic cavities.

Visceral peritoneum

The serous membrane that lines the surfaces of abdominal viscera. *Also see peritonitis.*

Visceral pleura

The serous membrane that lines the lung surfaces. *Also see pleural cavity.*

Visual agnosia

Inability to recognize the meaning of objects from visual cues.

Vital Capacity

See forced vital capacity.

Vitamins

Water-soluble or fat-soluble organic molecules present in foods. They are essential, in small amounts, for normal growth and for important metabolic functions. *Also see fat soluble vitamins.*

Vitreous humor

The clear gelatinous substance that occupies the space between the lens and retina. *Also see aqueous humor.*

W

Warfarin

An orally active coumarin anticoagulant. It acts by inhibiting vitamin K synthesis and depletion of the vitamin-K dependent clotting factors. May also be administered parenterally. It has significant interactions with other drugs and is a recognized teratogen. *Also see anticoagulation.*

Weber Test

A test, used along with Rinne's test, to distinguish conductive deafness from sensorineural hearing loss. It is performed by placing the stem of a vibrating tuning fork on the forehead and asking the patient to indicate in which ear the tone is louder. More advanced electronic audiologic tests are now commonly used for diagnosing hearing impairment. *Also see Rinne's test and deafness.*

Wernicke's area

The area of the parietal and temporal lobes of the left cerebral hemisphere that is responsible for speech recognition.

Western Blot

An analytical technique in which blot-immobilized target antigens are used for the detection of specific proteins in a patient's sample. Some important applications of this test include: confirmatory test for HIV infection, bovine spongiform encephalopathy (mad cow disease), and Lyme disease.

Wheal

See Triple response.

White blood cells (WBC)

See Leukocytes.

White matter

Part of the central nervous system which constitutes the region deep into the cerebral cortex and the outer portion of the spinal cord; it is composed primarily of myelinated fiber tracts.

White muscle

Skeletal muscle fibers that have characteristic features when compared to red muscle. These include: Fewer mitochondria, powerful but short contractions, rapid ATP metabolism, and lactic acid accumulation. Also called *"fast-twitch"* fibers.

Withdrawal Reflex

A protective reflex in which excitation, in response to a noxious stimulus, activates motor neurons supplying ipsilateral flexor muscles producing limb withdrawal. The withdrawal reflex is associated with inhibition of motor neurons that innervate the extensor muscles of the limb (reciprocal inhibition) as well as activation of motor neurons supplying contralateral extensor muscles (crossed extensor reflex).

Wolff-Chaikoff Effect

The phenomenon by which high blood iodine levels inhibit the transport of iodide ions, against both a chemical and an electrical gradient (iodine pump), into the thyroid follicular epithelial cells. Iodide toxicity can therefore cause hypothyroidism, goiter, or myxedema. The occasional hypothyroidism seen in patients receiving the iodine-containing anti-arrhythmic amiodarone has been attributed to this effect. *Also see tetraiodothyronine (thyroxine).*

X

X chromosome — The differential sex chromosome carried by all female gametes and half the male gametes.

Xenon — An inert gas that has been shown to have some anesthetic effects.

Y

Y Cells (retinal)	One of the retinal ganglion cells; they respond to rapid changes in the visual image.
Y chromosome	One of the two male sex chromosomes; the genes of this chromosome are important for male sexual determination and development.
Yellow marrow	A type of lipid storage tissue found within bone cavities.

Z

Z Disks

Components of the myofibril; dark-staining structures located in the middle of each I band, clearly delineating the ends of each sarcomere. *Also see sarcomere.*

Zidovudine (AZT)

Oral antiviral drug used for the treatment of HIV infection. *Also see Helper T cells.*

Zona fasiculata

See adrenal cortex

Zona glomerulosa

See adrenal cortex

Zona reticularis

See adrenal cortex

Zygote

A fertilized ovum.

Zymogen

An inactive precursor of an enzyme; a proenzyme. It undergoes biochemical change and is converted to the active form. A good example is pepsinogen; it is converted to the active pepsin.

Appendix I

Cardiovascular and Oxygenation Parameters

PARAMETER		FORMULA	UNITS
CARDIAC OUTPUT (CO)	=	HEART RATE X STROKE VOLUME	$L.min^{-1}$
CARDIAC INDEX (CI)	=	$\dfrac{\text{CARDIAC OUTPUT}}{\text{BODY SURFACE AREA (BSA)}}$	$L.min^{-1}.m^{-2}$
STROKE VOLUME (SV)	=	$\dfrac{\text{CARDIAC OUTPUT}}{\text{HEART RATE}}$	$ml.beat^{-1}$
STROKE VOLUME INDEX (SVI)	=	$\dfrac{\text{CARDIAC INDEX}}{\text{HEART RATE}}$	$ml.beat^{-1}.m^{-2}$
LEFT VENTRICULAR STROKE WORK (LVSW)	=	SVI x MAP x 0.0144	$g.m.m^{-2}.beat^{-1}$
RIGHT VENTRICULAR STROKE WORK (RVSW)	=	SVI x MPAP x 0.0144	$g.m.m^{-2}.beat^{-1}$
SYSTEMIC VASCULAR RESISTANCE (SVR)	=	$\dfrac{\text{MAP - CVP}}{\text{CO}}$ x 80	$dyne.sec.cm^{-5}.m^{-2}$
PULMONARY VASCULAR RESISTANCE (PVR)	=	$\dfrac{\text{MPAP - PCWP}}{\text{CO}}$ x 80	$dyne.sec.cm^{-5}.m^{-2}$
ARTERIAL OXYGEN CONTENT (CaO2)	=	Hb x $\dfrac{S_aO_2}{100}$ x 1.34	$ml.dl^{-1}$
MIXED VENOUS OXYGEN CONTENT ($C_{\bar{v}}O_2$)		Hb x $\dfrac{S_{\bar{v}}O_2}{100}$ x 1.34	$ml.dl^{-1}$
OXYGEN EXTRACTION RATIO (OER) (25-30%)	=	$\dfrac{C_aO_2 - C_{\bar{v}}O_2}{C_aO_2}$	%
SHUNT FRACTION (Q_s/Q_T)	=	$\dfrac{C_cO_2 - C_aO_2}{C_cO_2 - C_{\bar{v}}O_2}$	%
OXYGEN DELIVERY (DO_2I)	=	CI x C_aO_2 x 10	$ml.min^{-1}.m^{-2}$
OXYGEN CONSUMPTION (VO_2I)	=	CI x ($C_aO_2 - C_{\bar{v}}O_2$) x 10	$ml.min^{-1}.m^{-2}$

Note: For indexed SVR and PVR, use CI as the denominator

CPSIA information can be obtained at www.ICGtesting.com
Printed in the USA
238611LV00001B/1/P